FAMILY MEDICINE: A NEW APPROACH TO HEALTH CARE

The *Marriage & Family Review* series:

- *Family Medicine: A New Approach to Health Care,* edited by Betty E. Cogswell and Marvin B. Sussman
- *Cults & the Family,* edited by Florence Kaslow and Marvin B. Sussman
- *Alternatives to Traditional Family Living: An Update,* edited by Harriet Gross and Marvin B. Sussman
- *Ethnic Intermarriage in the United States,* edited by Gary A. Cretser and Joseph J. Leon

FAMILY MEDICINE: A NEW APPROACH TO HEALTH CARE

Betty E. Cogswell, Co-Editor
Marvin B. Sussman, Co-Editor

Volume 4, Numbers 1/2, Spring/Summer 1981
Marriage & Family Review

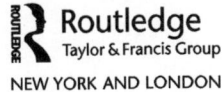

NEW YORK AND LONDON

Marriage & Family Review is published quarterly in the Spring, Summer, Fall, and Winter. Articles in this journal are selectively indexed or abstracted in: *The Chicago Psychoanalytic Literature Index, Psychological Abstracts,* and the *Psych/INFO* data base.

First published 1982 by The Haworth Press, Inc.

This edition published 2013 by Routledge

605 Third Avenue, New York, NY 10017
2 Park Square, Milton Park, Abingdon, Oxon OX14 4RN

Routledge is an imprint of the Taylor & Francis Group, an informa business

Library of Congress Cataloging in Publication Data
Main entry under title:

Family medicine, a new approach to health care.

(Marriage & family review, ISSN 0149-4929; v. 4, no. 1/2)
Includes bibliographies.
Contents: Family physician / Betty E. Cogswell -- The rise of family medicine / Donald C. Ransom -- Family medicine and holistic health / Kris Jeter -- [etc.]
1. Family medicine--Addresses, essays, lectures. I. Cogswell, Betty E. II. Sussman, Marvin B. III. Series. [DNLM: 1. Family practice. W1 MA68C v. 4. no. 1/2 / W 89 F197]
R729.5.G4F35 616 81-6980
ISBN 0-917724-25-9 AACR2

ISBN 13: 978-0-917724-25-1 (hbk)

DOI: 10.4324/9781315060781

Family Medicine: A New Approach to Health Care

Marriage & Family Review
Volume 4, Numbers 1/2, Spring/Summer 1981

Part I: OVERVIEW

Family Physician: A New Role in Process of Development 1
Betty E. Cogswell

The Rise of Family Medicine: New Roles for Behavioral Science 31
Donald C. Ransom

Family Medicine and Holistic Health: An Analytic Essay 73
Kris Jeter

Part II: a. SOCIALIZATION

Going Through Medical School and Considering the Choice of Family Medicine: Prescription or Antidote? 81
Hans O. Mauksch
Edward Brent
J. Timothy Diamond
Susan Elder

Education for the Practice of Family Medicine 103
John P. Geyman

Part II: b. PHYSICIAN/PATIENT ROLE

The Comprehensive Family Medicine Training Program: Has Sociology Found a Place in Graduate Medical Education? 113
Barbara Howe
Perry S. Warren

The Relational Model in Family Practice 123
Lynn P. Carmichael
Joan S. Carmichael

The Consumer and Family Physician Relationship: Power, Autonomy, Compliance, and Negotiation 135
Morton M. Warner

The Discipline of Family Medicine 157
Collin Baker

Family Medicine in Canada 163
J. Ivan Williams

FAMILY MEDICINE: A NEW APPROACH TO HEALTH CARE

FAMILY PHYSICIAN: A NEW ROLE IN PROCESS OF DEVELOPMENT

Betty E. Cogswell, PhD

Introduction

Family physicians, the most recently recognized specialists in American medicine, are in the enigmatic situation of developing the occupational role which they simultaneously occupy. In 1969 the Council on Medical Education of the American Medical Association (AMA) formally approved family medicine as the 20th specialty. Both prior to and since this date the emergence of this new discipline has been heavily rooted in reforms to correct deficits in contemporary practices of patient care. Family physicians are dedicated to providing continuing, comprehensive, primary care to families. This approach is viewed as a corrective for the fragmented, episodic, highly bureaucratic, and technocratic care many patients now receive. Interwoven with family physicians' reform efforts are their concerns with establishing a firm position of status, influence, and academic respectability within the institutional structure of medicine. These two issues–reform and family medicine's position within medicine–have influenced and most likely will continue to influence the process of development of this new role.

This process of role development is more easily observed among academic physicians than among those in private practice. Academicians have taken leadership in attempting to conceptualize the nature of their field and to publish the results of these efforts. Their publications indicate that they have been continually assessing their role, codifying definitions, and taking cognizance of the changing position of their field within medicine. Academicians are also a source of role innovations which they in turn pass on through the educational process to future family physicians.

The paper is organized around two topics: the influence of reform and position on the development of the role of family physician, and the presen-

Dr. Cogswell is Associate Professor of Family Medicine at the University of North Carolina, Chapel Hill, NC 27514.

Marriage & Family Review, Vol. 4(1/2), Spring/Summer 1981

tation of an analytic model which describes some components of this new role. My comments on the emergence of the role of family physicians and speculation as to its future course are framed within the sociological approach of symbolic interaction—a theoretical approach amenable to the study of role development (Note 1).

Theoretical Assumptions Underlying Role Development

Even roles which have matured and become institutionalized are never static, for there are always changes over time, however slight. In order to approximate reality, developing roles must be analyzed from a process rather than a static frame of reference. The majority of investigators have shown little concern with development of professions through time; they have instead viewed occupations and occupational roles as more or less static (Note 2). Some, however, have dealt with the processes by which occupations arise, take form, or change. A small portion of these investigators deal with roles of medical professionals (Smith, 1955; Bucher, 1962; Bucher & Strauss, 1961, 1968; Cogswell & Weir, 1964). Their studies focus on diversity and transformations within professional groups and the processes involved in their development.

Sociologists who analyze occupations as processes tend to have roots in the "Chicago" or symbolic interaction school of sociology (Note 3). This theoretical orientation leads one to focus on change over time, the variety of different perspectives within a profession, and the processes of continuous interactions which structure group life. Further, those who subscribe to this theoretical approach argue that highly structured human association is relatively infrequent and that institutionalized patterns constitute only a loose framework for daily behavior.

Particularly since the field of family medicine and the role of family physician are emergent, a symbolic interaction approach seems most appropriate as the basis for comment in this paper. Symbolic interaction points to the variety of perspectives among family physicians and individuals in other groups with whom family physicians continually interact and who together influence the definitional process. Processes of role definition proceed through family physicians' interactions and negotiations with each other and with patients, physicians in other medical specialties, paraprofessionals, hospital administrators, deans of medical schools, officials in state and federal governments, and members of the public at large.

Role definitions of family physician vary considerably both among family physicians and among people with whom they interact. Some individuals, particularly other medical specialists, see family medicine as merely another name for general practice. For others, family medicine is synonymous with primary care. This second definition prevails among many specialists and perhaps with less frequency among some state and federal officials, deans of medical schools, and hospital administrators. Although all family physicians would agree that they give primary care, they usually augment this definition to include delivery of continuing and comprehensive care. A large proportion of family physicians further elaborate their role to include emphasis on personalized and humanized care. A smaller group adds a third component to their role: caring for families. The largest proportion who subscribe to this last notion refer to family physicians' treating all members of a family. Others view patients within a family context where families are seen either as support groups for patients or as contributors to the etiology of disease. A few family physicians conceptualize families as small biosocial systems and consider this family system the proper unit of care. Among patient populations and the public at large, there are individuals who are likely to favor any one of the above definitions. Both the frequency and the degree to which family physicians and role relevant others subscribe to these definitions are matters for empirical research.

Family physicians speak of their specialty as one of breadth. They are generalists who primarily draw their scientific medicine and technical expertise from five older specialties–internal medicine, pediatrics, surgery, obstetrics-gynecology, and psychiatry-neurology. Compared to these specialties, family medicine is still a young field marked both by rapid expansion and by change, variety, ambiguity, and conflict in the images and definitions of the role of family physician. The reforms they champion require innovation; and, as has been pointed out, "Innovation...rests upon ambiguous, confused, not wholly defined situations" (Strauss, 1959, p. 26). It is in areas of ambiguity that transformations take place (Burke, 1945, p. 24) and new values and models for behavior emerge. Compared with older specialties, where roles are relatively static and their practitioners experience a rather quiet milieu, the definitional process of a new medical specialty is filled with exciting and dangerous experiences (Strauss, 1959, p. 144). Individual and collective actions by family physicians are still tentative and exploratory, and it is likely that both the ends of and the means to role development will be reformulated as the role evolves.

Influence of Reform and Position on Role Development

A growing awareness of the need for reforms in patient care has stemmed from two major sources: the medical profession itself and critics in the society at large. Family physicians have addressed reforms as a basis for establishing a new specialty and for determining the goals for role development. At this point, family physicians are better able to articulate what they want to improve in the present system of medical care than to state the exact nature of their specialty and the means by which they hope to correct these deficits. The desire to attain a respected and influential position within the field of medicine also influences family physicians' image of their role, the nature of their reform efforts, and the speed with which these reforms can be implemented within their own specialty.

The Need for a Reform Movement in Patient Care

The reaction of the medical profession to the Flexner Report published in 1910 and the resulting reorganization of medical education which led to a proliferation of medical specialties in the following decades are often cited as the causes of the need for reforms in medicine today. Prior to this report, most of the physicians in the United States were general practitioners who provided the majority, if not all, of the care for their patients, seeing them on a continuing basis as needed over a lifetime (Note 4).

> The general practitioner of revered memory knew his patients, did whatever he could to cure or ease their varied ailments, and provided continuing care through the course of minor ailments and major emergencies. His deficiencies–and they were many–were partly offset by intimate knowledge of his patients, the support he gave them, and the trust and confidences his services engendered (Millis, 1966, p. 33).

Concerned about the quality of care and the inadequacy of medical training, Flexner advocated higher standards and longer periods of graduate training. Eventually, medical schools and residency programs graduated more specialists and fewer physicians trained for primary care. Specialists tended to locate their practices in urban medical centers where they could have access to advanced technology, supportive services, and consultations from other specialists. As a result, rural areas were underserved and patient care became highly bureaucratic, technocratic, fragmented, and episodic. Family medicine is a response both to correcting these deficiencies and preserving the assets of general practitioners: a 3-year residency program provides a more adequate grounding in scientific medicine than general practitioners receive, and reforms in the delivery of patient care correct for medicine's overreaction to the Flexner report.

Awareness within medicine of need for reform. In the 1960s some segments within the medical establishment became concerned about medicine's neglect of quality primary care and recognized the need for establishing a primary care specialty with a solid position in institutionalized medicine and medical education. In 1966 three separate blue ribbon commissions published reports which ushered in family medicine, charting a course for its formal establishment and launching it on a mission of reform [*The Graduate Education of Physicians: The Report of the Citizens' Commission on Graduate Medical Education* (The Millis Report); *Health Services* (The Folsom Report); *Meeting the Challenge of Family Practice: The Report of the Ad Hoc Committee on Education for Family Practice* (The Willard Report).] The authors of all three reports speak of the need in American medicine to overcome barriers to providing continuing and comprehensive patient care, and they express concern about geographic maldistribution of physicians and the decreasing ratio of primary care physicians to medical specialists. In each report there is a strong affirmation that individuals and families throughout the country should have easy access to personal physicians oriented toward the whole person and providing both scientific medicine and humanistic care.

Societal criticisms of established medicine. Family medicine originated and has continued to grow during a period of social unrest in which there has been a growing disenchantment with and a call for reform of the established system of medical care. Criticisms have come from many sources and have taken a variety of forms, ranging from radical indictments to more moderate but critical appraisals. Ivan Illich (1975), in a sweeping accusation, begins *Medical Nemesis* with the sentence, "The medical establishment has become a major threat to health" (p. 11). Illich goes on to describe iatrogenesis (physician/hospital-inflicted illness) as rampant in today's medical system. Similar protests are made by some feminists identified with the women's health movement (Corea, 1977; Frankfort, 1972; Ehrenreich & English, 1973). Somewhat less severe criticisms come from patients, many concerned physicians, and the public at large, who are disturbed about the health negating consequences of overmedication, excessive surgery, excessive reliance on technology, overbureaucratization, and the shift of health care from the community to the medical center. Influential critics like Senator Edward Kennedy (1972) and other spokesmen for federal and state governments are concerned about the cost of care and the unavailability of care for many segments of our population, such as minority groups, the poor, and rural residents. It should be noted that these criticisms center around the practice of medicine—the application of scientific knowledge and techniques to patient care—and are not criticisms of scientific medical knowledge per se.

Family Medicine's Position Within Medicine

In response to criticisms of medical care both within medicine and from society at large, family medicine has recently made extraordinary advances. The field was approved as a clinical specialty, residency programs for training new members were established, two national organizations representing family physicians' interests were formed, and a refereed journal was begun. Even with these advances, many family physicians are still concerned with achieving a respected position within medicine. Some family physicians may merely want the additional prestige associated with other specialties, but the primary goal of others seems to be gaining the influence necessary to implement reforms within their own specialty and within medical education in general. The interrelationship between implementing reforms and establishing a more secure position within the field of medicine is a delicate question for family physicians (Carmichael, 1978) for reform has been the source of vitality for the family medicine movement, and this vitality could be lost in negotiations and compromises with established medicine (Stephens, 1976).

Indicators of an established position. In 1969 the Council on Medical Education of the American Medical Association (AMA) formally approved the specialty of family practice and recognized the American Board of Family Practice which is authorized to examine and certify physicians. The Board consisted of 15 members, five from the American Academy of General Practice, five from the Section on General Practice of the AMA, and one each from five specialty Boards–Surgery, Medicine, Pediatrics, Obstetrics-Gynecology, and Psychiatry-Neurology (Walsh, 1970). It is important to point out that the boards of the older specialties are composed entirely of members from their own specialty while the American Board of Family Practice includes one member from each of five other specialties. Family medicine draws from the clinical base of these five specialties in defining its scope of work. One can argue that representatives of these other specialties serve on the Board to assure clinical competence and expertise in their respective areas and to add prestige to board certification. Conversely, the presence of other specialists can be viewed by institutionalized medicine as a watchdog arrangement which reduces the professional autonomy of family physicians. One future indication that family medicine has proven itself to other specialties might be reconstitution of board membership to include only board certified family physicians.

The Board was charged to examine and certify three categories of candidates: (1) physicians who have completed a 3-year residency program in family practice, (2) those currently members of the American Academy of

General Practice who held recertification for membership by the Academy for 6 years, and (3) those who have been recertified by the Academy for the immediate past 3 years and, in addition, take two of several options of additional training. A unique provision for certification for this specialty is that there is no grandfather clause (no one is exempt from being examined) and that periodic recertification for board certified family physicians is required every year even for those completing a residency (Walsh, 1970). The larger proportion of currently certified family physicians have not completed a residency but rather have achieved that status through recertification. Availability of the recertification options for board eligibility without residency training may have lowered the prestige of family medicine in the eyes of other specialists. Since 1978, the only route to Board eligibility is through successfully completing a 3-year residence program in family medicine (Pisacano, 1978). As the ranks of the specialty become filled with a higher and higher proportion of residency-trained physicians, the field may achieve greater prestige within medicine.

Since 1969, residency programs have grown at an astronomical rate. In 1970, there were five family medicine residency programs in the United States, and by 1978 there were 348 (American Academy of Family Physicians, 1978). Approximately 16% of these residencies are university based, 12% community based and university administered, and 50% community based and university affiliated. The other 22% are either community based and unaffiliated or are programs in the military (American Academy of Family Physicians, 1978). By 1978, 106 (81%) of the 131 medical schools in the United States had active departments, divisions, or programs in family medicine (Phillips, 1978).

Other indicators of institutionalization appeared during the same period. In 1968, the Society of Teachers of Family Medicine was formed in anticipation of the approval of residency programs. Membership in this society is open to all faculty members in family medicine programs and includes behavioral and social scientists in addition to physicians. Inclusion of nonphysician members indicates a recognition of the contributions of other fields in the training of family physicians. In 1971, the American Academy of General Practice changed its name to the American Academy of Family Physicians (Bruce, 1973). In 1974, the *Journal of Family Practice* became the first refereed journal in family medicine although there were several nonrefereed predecessors.

Continuing concern about position. Despite these advances, family medicine has a relatively insecure position within medical education and has not achieved the status, influence, and academic respectability of other specialties.

Even after the specialty was formally acknowledged by institutionalized medicine, family physicians have experienced a variety of negative responses from medical colleagues in other specialties. Carmichael (1978) perceived three stages in the reactions of those in medicine to family medicine: first, the field was ignored; second, it was actively opposed; and now, family medicine is entering a third stage of possible co-optation by medicine. Carmichael warns family physicians to resist this third stage. He sees co-optation as an immoral option which would retard family medicine's reform efforts.

Negative reactions within medicine might be attributed to a variety of reasons, each of which requires empirical investigation. One reason may be opposition by some segments in medicine to the reforms family physicians champion. Another reason may include the lower status attributed to general medicine in relation to specialized medicine. Most other specialties are based on an in-depth expertise discretely defined by a body system (e.g., cardiology), gender of the patient (e.g., obstetrics-gynecology), age of the patient (e.g., pediatrics), or on technological advances (e.g., radiology). In contrast, family physicians' claim to technical expertise is a generalist role, broadly based on a number of other specialties. There is, moreover, a lack of academic experience among family medicine faculty, who were recruited from clinical practice and had to learn the basics of teaching, academic politics, and educational administration. In addition, most of these practitioners have no background in research and publication—two mandatory achievements for advancement in academic settings. Furthermore, family physicians are criticized by other specialists for their inability to state the exact nature of their role and expertise. Finally, there may be resentment from some segments of the medical profession that family medicine's primary mandate for formation and growth can be attributed to pressures by state and federal government and to consumers (Pelligrino, 1978; Walton, 1977).

Leaders in the field of medicine may have underestimated the importance of the public's needs and point of view during the rush toward specialization and thus neglected corrective measures. Freidson (1970), in a sociological analysis of the medical profession, emphasizes the importance of the lay public to the establishment and continuation of any consulting/practicing profession. In tracing the history of medicine, Freidson notes that over the past century medicine gained prestige and an organized autonomy which permitted it to develop its own institutions for serving public needs. These institutions became increasingly independent of the public and were organized according to professional rather than lay standards. Maintaining such distance from the lay public permitted enormous advances in scientific knowledge and technique but eroded previous advances in the practice of medicine.

> It is precisely in applying knowledge to human affairs...where extensive professional autonomy is justified neither morally nor professionally. It is not justified morally...human beings, even if laymen, have a right to determine what their own problems are and to have a voice in how they are to be managed. It is not justified functionally...because it leads the profession to be blind to its own shortcomings and unable to regulate its practices adequately (Freidson, 1970, p. 371).

Family physicians believe that they take much greater cognizance than other specialists of the desires and needs of the lay public, and in particular of their patients/consumers. Attention to consumerism is woven into family physicians' styles of practice through their commitment to the role of patient advocate (Stephens, 1976). Social validation and support from the public for the role of family physician is likely to increase with family physicians' implementation of reforms. If family physicians become the primary medical contact for an increasingly larger proportion of the patient population and if they, in partnership with patients, become the decision makers about referrals to other specialists, it is possible that the tide may turn and family physicians may eventually become the watchdogs of other specialists. Perhaps with strong support from the lay public, family physicians can maintain their commitment to reform and also gain influence and respect within the medical establishment.

Family physicians, trained in scientific medicine and dedicated to an agenda of reform, attempt to bridge the value systems of both medicine and the lay society. This dual value system may account in part for the problems family physicians are experiencing in developing a role acceptable to themselves, the public, and the medical establishment.

An Analytic Model of the Role of Family Physician

Family physicians are drawing from many sources in their attempts to develop innovative models of patient care. Because family medicine is a specialty within organized medicine, it is logical to expect family physicians to draw from medicine those definitions which they find compatible with their emerging role. Since many definitions within established medicine are incompatible, selection requires careful consideration. The goals posited by the three blue ribbon commissions are embraced by family physicians, but these goals provide only general guidelines, and the tasks of working out the details are still in progress. Knowledge and theoretical approaches in the social and behavioral sciences show promise but usually require translation from the general to the specific to be of immediate relevance for practice. The perspectives of the lay public and of patients are important to family physicians, but these perspectives are variable and often have not been clearly expressed.

However, with the rise of consumer movements and the women's health movement, the public is becoming more articulate and more assertive about specific needs and desires concerning the delivery of care. Tailoring patient care to patients' needs has become essential to the formation of the role of the family physician.

Stephens (1975), a family physician, presents the thesis that "patient management is the quintessential skill of clinical practice and the unique field of knowledge of family physicians" (p. 423), "and is the intellectual and academic basis for family practice" (p. 428). "Patient management" is a narrower concept than "practice" or "patient care" but is an important aspect of those activities (Note 5). Stephens sees concentration of attention on this issue as the primary route for family physicians to advance beyond the ambiguities and confusions inherent in the field today toward a clearer definition of their role and their field. In this paper the term "patient management" is replaced with the term "styles of practice" which includes Stephens' concept but is much broader.

Family physicians' development of new approaches to patient care is an uneven process; some of their goals are defined more fully and are integrated more completely into practice than others. In addition, different interest groups within the field of family medicine have contributed toward clarifying goals, each making distinct choices and proceeding at varying rates to incorporate those goals into their ideology and practice. It is important to keep these variations in mind in considering the analytic model which follows.

The analytic model of the role of family physician presented in this paper reflects the ideologies of academic family physicians and is viewed as a hypothetical basis for describing current practice and future developments in the field. Even in this setting, wide variation in ideology and practice rather than a monolithic situation is to be expected. The model of this role has three main components:

1. *Delivery of continuing, comprehensive, primary care* which requires changes in the organizational structure of the present system of health care delivery.

2. *Emphasis on the human dimensions of medicine* which are evolving as a result of reordering value priorities of established medicine.

3. *Focus on the family rather than the individual* as the appropriate unit of medical care.

Although development is continually occurring within all three components of this role, some analytic advantages are gained by viewing these components as forming a logical sequence. Continuing, comprehensive care is necessary if physicians are to develop a humanized approach with relationships of trust, empathy, and intimacy with patients (Walton, 1977)—relationships which in turn enable physicians to focus on families instead of individuals.

Viewing these three components sequentially permits the presentation of some working hypotheses. Each succeeding role component is:

1. less clearly defined,
2. less standardized,
3. less frequently implemented in practice,
4. more apt to be derived from sources outside the medical profession, and
5. more apt to differentiate family medicine from other specialties.

The intent here is to present a conceptual scheme as a guide to ordering new styles of practice emerging in family medicine. The reader should be warned, however, that this conceptualization of the role of family physician will need to be modified or replaced as family physicians continue to develop role definitions. Statements made in the following discussion of the three role components require empirical investigation to determine both the exact nature of definitions and the degree to which definitions have been incorporated into behavior by different segments within family medicine. Statements comparing family medicine to other medical specialties also require empirical verification.

A New Organizational Structure to Provide Continuing, Comprehensive Care by Primary Physicians

The three blue-ribbon commissions envisioned family physicians as "horizontal specialists" who can deal with the large majority of patients' needs on a continuing basis (Note 6) and envisioned this role as integrating humanized care with a high level of competence in scientific medicine. The emerging curricula of family practice residency programs are intended to attain these goals. In contrast to the training of the general practitioner, the additional training that family physicians receive is intended to make them more proficient generalists in scientific medicine and more humanistic clinicians through formal training in appropriate interpersonal skills and in the behavioral and social sciences. Implementation of this role, however, requires reorganization within the medical system (Folsom, 1966), for continuing, comprehensive care by primary physicians is difficult if not impossible within the normative organizational structures of highly specialized medical centers.

The two concepts, *continuing* care and *comprehensive* care, developed within the medical system and were a part of the medical vocabulary long before the advent of family medicine. Physicians, however, disagree about the meanings of these terms, and changes in definition have taken place over time. The most straightforward meaning of continuing care is that patients repeatedly see the same group of physicians. This contact is augmented by a single well-kept medical chart which provides knowledge of previous problems and treatments. Curtis and Rogers (1978) review the literature on continuity of care and note variations in definitions. In addition, they attempt to describe an evolving consensus about the term occurring among family physicians.

> Most commentators in the field of Family Medicine, as well as some in Pediatrics, contend that continuity is exemplified by the feeling of the physician which embodies a continuing and caring responsibility for the person and the family rather than concern about specific problems per se. It appears that this feeling of personal responsibility (even after regular office hours) grows, as continuity of care improves. It has also been suggested that the patient must accept certain responsibilities to maintain the "continuity contract." McWhinney notes that the nature of this contract is a central issue for family medicine and "is terminated only by mutual agreement, or by decision of one of the parties" (p. 122).

The concept comprehensive care perhaps has wider variations in meaning. Somers, a medical economist, notes that "comprehensive care is basically a philosophical concept, about whose precise meaning reasonable men will continue to differ" (1968). To some physicians comprehensive care simply means the medical tasks of a generalist to treat 85% to 95% of patients' illnesses (Lynn, 1977). The blue-ribbon reports and most family physicians add to this definition by providing a wide array of care including preventive, health maintenance, rehabilitative, health education, psychological, social, and counseling services. Gordis and Markowitz (1971) extend the meaning of comprehensive into the realm of continuing care by adding that comprehensive care requires that the physician be continuously available to patients in person and by phone beyond clinic hours so that patients also have access to their physicians at night and on weekends.

Reorganization in the medical system necessary to the delivery of continuing, comprehensive care is beginning to occur. The establishment and rapid growth of family medicine residency programs is taking place. Family physicians have begun to develop new organizational structures for teaching and practice which are different from those of other specialties. Organizational changes can be described briefly in terms of four themes which are closely interrelated with family physicians' expressed values.

1. *Integration Rather than Continuing Differentiation.* Family medicine represents a shift away from medicine's trend toward increasing role differentiation through specialization which has contributed to episodic, fragmented care. Family physicians are generalists who incorporate many technical functions within a single role. Thus, a single physician can care for most problems that patients present. When a problem is beyond a family physician's expertise the patient will be referred to an appropriate specialist. Even then, most family physicians continue to remain in constant contact with the patient and the other physician. Furthermore, family physicians are trained to give care to all age groups from birth to death. Integration of this wide assortment of medical care into one role potentially permits greater humanization of care, and this continuing physician/patient relationship becomes analogous to relationships within the family—the group par excellence which performs undifferentiated functions.

2. *Decentralization: Community-Based Medical Care.* Family physicians tend to practice alone, in partnership, or in small groups and tend to locate their offices in communities rather than in hospital medical centers. In contrast to other specialists, family physicians are geographically and bureaucratically more accessible to their patients, and are thus more likely to see their patients on a continuing basis and are more apt to be knowledgeable about the families, neighborhoods, and communities they serve.

3. *Relational Style: A Shift from Authoritarian to Colleague Roles.* An authoritarian structure is often considered the hallmark of medicine. In comparison, some family physicians have embraced a much more democratic style in small organizations such as group practices, residency training programs, and medical school departments. Concurrently, among family physicians, one sees changes in traditional superordinate and subordinate role relationships between physician and patient, between physician and other health care workers such as nurses and social workers, and between teacher and students. This is particularly important in relationships with patients in which physicians have traditionally been paternalistic and authoritarian.

4. *Scale: Small Is Beautiful.* As specialization in medicine led to greater dependence of specialists upon each other and to the use of increasingly sophisticated, expensive medical equipment, there was a rapid growth of large medical centers (Millis, 1966, p. 92). Thus, patients seeking care were faced

with large-scale, impersonal bureaucracies. Ideally and in practice family medicine emphasizes "small scale" which in turn is associated with "human scale." Even in residency training programs located in large teaching hospitals, family practice centers are organized to minimize bureaucracy. Centers have their own patient registrations and appointment services separated from those of the medical center. Patient charts are maintained in the family practice center rather than in a centralized hospital chart room. Practice teams often are organized so that the same receptionist, nurse, social worker, and physician see a given panel of patients. Space is arranged and decorated to resemble a small office in an attempt to achieve a personal rather than a sterile atmosphere. Efforts are made to assure easy parking and physical accessibility.

Summary. It may be useful to summarize this discussion in terms of the five working hypotheses about the components of the role mentioned previously. The development of an organizational structure necessary to give continuing, comprehensive care is the most highly developed and institutionalized component of family physicians' current style of practice. Family practitioners are much clearer about this component of their role than about the following two components and have incorporated it into practice and education throughout the country. Even though continuing, comprehensive care is posited as a corrective to the episodic, fragmented care of established medicine, these concepts are drawn from the field of medicine. Only the degree of emphasis on continuing, comprehensive care differentiates family medicine from many other specialties, but this emphasis does little to differentiate it from the large number of internists and pediatricians who deliver primary care. One distinction even here is that internists treat only adults and pediatricians only children, while family practitioners care for patients of all ages from birth to death and are thereby able to care for all members of a family.

Values: Attempts to Humanize Scientific Medicine

Humanized care is valued throughout medicine; however, in many quarters it has lower priority in the value hierarchy than considerations such as technical competence with sophisticated diagnostic and treatment techniques, demonstration of highly specialized knowledge about a limited domain, and treatment of diseases rather than people. Although there is a sizable body of literature on the humanization of medical care, readers find it obvious that the field is in a state of conceptual chaos (Mechanic, 1975). Definitions are inadequate, and there is a tendency to address issues of dehumanization rather than humanization. Geiger (1975), a physician and professor of community medicine, comments on this orientation.

> I am more comfortable defining the task of identifying dehumanization and fighting it, rather than identifying humanization and supporting it. This says something either about my training as a physician, with its massive emphasis on identifying and treating pathology, or about my personal emotional bent toward finding pathology and fighting it, or both" (p. 12).

Some of the most coherent commentaries on humanizing medicine are made by a group of writers representing a variety of disciplines and perspectives in a book edited by Howard and Strauss, entitled *Humanizing Health Care* (1975). Authors in this book emphasized four major causes of dehumanized health care: the impact of strict professionalism, the impact of modern technology, the increasing organizational size of health facilities, and the inequities in American life (Strauss, 1975, p. 227). A few of the authors in this volume attempt to deal with humanization. Howard (1975, p. 57-102) identifies eight necessary and sufficient conditions for humanized health care: inherent worth of human beings, irreplaceability of individuals, holistic selves, freedom of action, status equality, shared decision making and responsibility, empathy, and positive effect. These dimensions are described and illustrated with sufficient clarity to be useful as guidelines for physicians desiring to practice medicine in a more humanized manner and for investigators to classify but not measure physician/patient behavior.

The Institute for the Study of Humanistic Medicine has published several books of essays on humanized medicine (Blau et al., 1975; Remen et al., 1975; Miller et al., 1975). Authors of these publications are weak on conceptualization, relying heavily on case histories and vignettes to provide insights into dehumanized and humanized care. Remen (1975), a pediatrician, presents a more advanced conceptual scheme than the other authors in attempting to define humanized care. She emphasizes several basic principles: holism is preferable to reductionism; medicine is an art as well as a science; and colleagueship in physician/patient relationships is preferable to authoritarianism. These and other dimensions, however, are not sufficiently specified or illustrated to serve as a ready paradigm for either practice or research.

Although almost all family physicians would affirm that delivery of humanized medical care is an important component of their role, the lack of definition and conceptualization and the ensuing ambiguities make practice and teaching difficult. Considerable effort will be required to develop a sufficiently coherent approach to patient care and to teach this approach in an orderly fashion to residents and medical students.

Values Drawn from the Larger Society

Newly developing orientations in family medicine mirror values which have been emerging and are becoming pervasive in the larger society. Analysis of these societal values provides insight for developing new patterns of practice which are more humanistic than those currently offered by specialty medicine.

Family medicine emerged during a period of general challenge to existing institutions and established values in American society. The societal climate of the 1960s was conducive to innovation in very diverse areas of life, and medicine was no exception. The civil rights movement, the women's liberation movement, the antiwar movement, and the New Left advanced liberal or radical challenges to the "Establishment." The counterculture, a much more diffuse social phenomenon than the political movements, posed a more subtle but pervasive challenge to the status quo. Contemporary social movements had impact not only by creating a situation favorable for institutional changes, such as the rise of family medicine as a new medical specialty, but also by bringing about changes in societal values which paved the way for the emergence of the specific ideals that took root in the ideology of family medicine. Five values which have recently gained salience in the larger society (Note 7) and which family physicians are beginning to integrate into the physician/patient relationship in their daily practice are discussed below. It appears likely that family medicine has received and will receive support from those segments of the lay public who adhere to these values.

1. Search for community. Modern societies are characterized by the predominance of large-scale bureaucratic organizations which channel and sometimes control human behavior. Modernization has produced various undesirable consequences, such as alienation of individuals from the community, workers from the tools and product of work, and family members from each other. Different groups have sought in different ways to escape isolation and loneliness. The alternate culture of the 1960s attempted to create instant kinship and utopian communities as refuges from society. Others attempted to counter loneliness through revival of ethnic identities, preservation of urban neighborhoods, and search for family roots.

The ideology of family medicine parallels, in at least two important ways, the theme of search for community. First, whereas many specialties are oriented toward treating a diseased organ or organ system, family physicians stress treating the human being as a unit of biological, psychological, and social functions. The notion of family as the unit of health reflects a view of the human being as a member of primary groups and communities rather than as a social atom. Second, family physicians express a search for community in their attempt to insure that the relationship between patient and physician is a personal one, as befits members of a community. Indeed, some family physicians consider that the adjective *family* in the title of the specialty refers to the nature of the patient-doctor relationship (Carmichael, 1976). Curry (1977) has more modestly argued that family physicians need to reexamine the concept of professional distance, noting that they can feel compassion and empathy toward their patients without distorting the professional relationship.

Search for community has appeal for both practitioners and patients. As a career, family medicine offers an opportunity to those who want to avoid entanglement in medical center bureaucracies and who seek to help "real" people, yet want a prestigious and remunerative occupation. Likewise, family physicians appeal to consumers who resent being treated "like a number" or "as another case." In effect, they attract patients who react against having their illnesses managed as bureaucratic problems, but who still want the benefits of modern medical science. Thus, one finds both a ready supply of recruits into family medicine and a market for their services.

2. Rise in tolerance of alternative lifestyles. Compared to the 1950s and 1960s, tolerance of "alternative life-styles" is considerably greater today, despite more recent resurgence of limits to tolerance as the conservative groups mobilize to repeal laws legalizing abortions, repeal "gay rights" ordinances, and fight passage of the Equal Rights Amendment. During the last decade society has seen an increase in the number of, as well as acceptance of, unmarried, childless, and homosexual couples, as well as voluntary singles and divorced persons (Cogswell & Sussman, 1972). The traditional nuclear family, with father as the sole breadwinner and mother at home raising the children, considered the predominant family form since industrialization began, now constitutes only 13% of American families (Ramey, 1978). In short, more people today live in arrangements different from the traditional nuclear family and find greater societal tolerance of these arrangements. To the extent that many human service systems–health, education, and welfare–have based their policies and practices on the image of the traditional nuclear family, they have diminished the value and appropriateness of their services and have often worked to the detriment of many of the individuals and families they are attempting to serve. (See Cogswell, 1975; Cogswell & Sussman, 1972, for a more complete explanation.)

Many family physicians have manifested this societal value of tolerance of alternative life-styles by stressing a nonjudgmental approach toward all types of patients, by attempting to integrate patients' life situations into day-to-day clinical practice, and by adopting broad definitions of family. "The term family (in family medicine) is used in the broadest sense to describe any group of intimates with a history and a future" (Ransom & Vandervoort, 1973).

3. Back to nature. The rise of environmentalism, the ecology movement, the increase in the popularity of natural foods and organic farming, the rebirth of crafts, and the proliferation of natural approaches to health can be cited as manifestations of a move back to nature. As Dubos (1959) has pointed out, just as "the natural state" has been seen as utopian where social life is concerned, the "way of nature" has been equated through the ages with good health.

In recent years medicine has been accused by the public of overmedicating patients, performing unnecessary surgery, and using sophisticated diagnostic techniques routinely rather than only when warranted. Family physicians, on the other hand, tend to favor use of the least intrusive diagnostic and therapeutic techniques appropriate to the patient's condition and have been at the forefront in reassessing the costs, dangers, and benefits of procedures. In treatment, family physicians appear less likely than other specialists to immediately prescribe medication or surgery for problems, recognizing that some problems can be treated effectively with natural approaches such as exercise, diet, rest, or changes in life-style. Extensive diagnostic work-ups are not routine for all patients; rather, family physicians carefully assess both the financial and health costs and proceed cautiously (Note 8). Family physicians' emphasis on prevention and on the social and psychological dimensions of health and illness are also consistent with their moderation in the use of sophisticated technology. In addition, the use of drugs as palliatives is discouraged in cases where the source of the complaint is primarily social or psychological. Instead, a search for the real source of the complaint and intervention at the social or psychological level is recommended.

In sum, family physicians stress natural approaches to patient care. Emphasis on the natural leads to increased awareness of and contraindictions for excesses in the use of drugs, sophisticated procedures, and advanced technology and leads to progressive, gradual approaches in treatment.

4. Struggle for equality. In the last three decades, blacks, the poor, students, women, and minorities have become aware of certain social inequities and deprivations and have fought for equal status in American society. Within this context, the traditional doctor-patient relationship which tends to be a superordinate/subordinate role has come under strong criticism (Waitzkin & Waterman, 1974). Some observers argue that inequality in the doctor/patient relationship is inevitable given the inherent gap in relevant knowledge and competence (e.g., Parsons, 1975). Others point out that the potential for exploitation always exists when such inequalities are present and emphasize that the degree of inequality in the relationship can vary with the nature of the medical situation, the psychological makeup of the participants, and the social characteristics of the patients (Szasz & Hollender, 1956).

Family physicians advance a more egalitarian model of the doctor/patient relationship than is typical in modern medicine. This is in keeping with their emphasis on patient education, which tends to decrease the knowledge gap between physician and patient. Furthermore, family physicians appear to be giving patients more power in the role relationship by presenting alternative diagnostic and treatment procedures and the expected outcomes and consequences of each, so that patients may choose among medically acceptable alternatives. When the entire family is involved in the therapeutic relationship, the power differential between physician and patient may be reduced further, because patients do not have to face the authority figure of the physician in isolation but potentially may receive support from other family members.

5. Personal growth (and self-actualization). The Protestant ethic of success, defined as individual achievement in the occupational world, was, if not eroded by the values of the alternate culture of the 1960s, at least supplemented with an ethic of psychological and emotional growth and the requirement to experience the world, not merely succeed in it. Activities ranging from meditation to jogging are seen as promoting "growth" and enhancing the physical, psychological, and spiritual self. In medicine the counterpart of the concept of personal growth is the emphasis on defining health positively—as something to be systematically worked for and enhanced, rather than as the mere absence of pathology. Such a conception of health is generally compatible with family physicians' insistence on preventive and continuing care and on health education; moreover, it leads family physicians to consider patients as active participants in their own health maintenance.

Summary. To humanize medical care, family physicians are attempting to reorder priorities within medicine and incorporate values from the larger society. Current definitions and behavioral implications of humanized care are less specific than those of continuing and comprehensive care. Within the medical system, almost all physicians would favor humanized care; but many give only lip service to this goal and other values often assume precedence as guides to behavior. Family physicians, however, appear to be making a collective effort to define and implement a style of practice which humanizes medical care. Family physicians' special emphasis on humanized care gives them the potential for achieving styles of practice very different from those currently institutionalized in specialty medicine.

Family: As the Unit of Health Care

By the name alone, *family* medicine and *family* practice emphasize that this is a medical specialty concerned with families. Among family physicians, however, differences of opinion exist about the meaning and importance of family as the unit of care. Some proponents emphasize that treating families rather than individuals is the major focus of family physicians' style of practice and the major issue which distinguishes family medicine from other medical specialties (Carmichael, 1966; Olsen, 1970; Worby, 1971; Geyman & Hawkes, 1973; Ransom & Vandervoort, 1973; Mauksch, 1974). Others who recognize the urgent need for continuing, comprehensive, primary care delivered in a humanistic manner tend to neglect the family in an attempt to realize these goals (Pellegrino, 1978).

Even among those who insist that treating families is a vital issue for family medicine, there are no clear statements as to how this is done. Exactly what is implied by designating the family as the unit of care requires clarification both in theory and in practice. Carmichael (1966) has written that "family medicine is the branch of medical science that has as its responsibility the continuing health maintenance of the family." He views the family in the sociological sense as the basic unit in society, the "unit of living." It is clear that the intent here is beyond the notion that a single family physician attends each family member. Minimally, it means that clinicians must take the family into account as an important variable when dealing with an individual patient (Bruce, 1973). Family physicians must understand the role of the family in the promotion and maintenance of health (Pratt, 1976), in the etiology of disease (Note 9), and in adjustment of the family group to illness and disability of one of its members (Cogswell, 1975).

Social scientists have taken leadership in considering families' influence on health and illness; however, their work to date offers only partial guidance to family physicians. Ransom (1981) in this special issue of *Marriage & Family Review*, highlights the importance of a family-centered approach to health care. Litman (1974) has prepared the most comprehensive review of the literature to date, citing over 1,000 references on the family as a basic unit in health and medical care. In summarizing the state of the field, Litman notes, "First and foremost, there is a need for greater application and integration of family theory in health care research" (1974, p. 510). Few investigators have given attention to the role of the family in individual illness or the effect of illness on family life (Vincent, 1963). "Such major issues as familiar response, adjustment, and behavior in health and illness have generally escaped the empirical involvement and theoretical interest of the family sociologist" (Litman, 1974, p. 495). Further, medical sociologists who investigate these issues focus on individuals and seldom study families. Practitioners' use of family as a unit of care requires synthesis of existing theory and knowledge about family and health and requires new investigations combining the two approaches. Advancement is further hampered by family sociologists' inattention to conceptualizing and studying families as small social systems (Hill, 1974). Theories of family groups are not sufficiently advanced for immediate application in either medical practice or research. If family physicians and social scientists were to join in interdisciplinary efforts, their work should provide more realistic and relevant guidelines for clinical care of families.

Treating family as patient requires both a conceptual and a behavioral shift from established patterns in medicine today. It is perhaps useful both to identify and to place family in a context of other units of care. Viewing the entire field of medicine, I have abstracted seven ways of conceptualizing units of care and have presented them in order of increasingly larger units:

1. *An organ system*, such as circulatory, neurological, and female reproductive systems which are units of care of specific medical specialties.
2. *Human as biological organism*, the unit of scientific medicine.
3. *Human as an individual*, the unit of scientific, humanized medicine.
4. *Individual in family context*, in which the patient is an individual but family influences on etiology, treatment, and recovery are taken into account. This model is used frequently by family physicians, psychiatrists, and, occasionally, by other specialists.
5. *Family group conceptualized as a sum total of individuals* is an additive model which is exemplified by family physicians treating each individual member of a family.
6. *Family group conceptualized as a small biosocial system* is an innovative approach which a few family physicians, other physicians, and social scientists are attempting to develop.
7. *Community*, the traditional unit of practice for public health and community medicine.

It is important to investigate the frequency with which each unit is used in practice by physicians in different specialties.

Within the field of family medicine there is wide variation both in theory and practice as to the appropriate unit of care. Indeed, as the field develops we may find that the relevant unit logically depends on the reason the patient seeks medical care and the immediate and long-range circumstances surrounding this event. The appropriate unit of care for a person experiencing cardiac arrest might be the organ system at first, but as care continues the appropriate units might be the individual, the individual in family context, and the family group. As this illustration points out, what is needed is not just a rhetoric extolling the use of a single unit of care, but rather a specification of criteria indicating which unit is most relevant at a given moment for a given set of circumstances. For the relevant unit to be used, however, physicians must be trained and competent to practice with the range of possibilities and no lesser unit should be used when a more expanded unit is appropriate. Thus, it is important to be able to conceptualize and deal with the following units: the individual in family context, the family as a sum total of individuals, and the family as a biosocial system. In developing methods for practicing with these three units, family medicine could make a major contribution to medical care.

Family Conceptualized as a Sum Total of Individuals. This approach is perhaps the easiest to conceptualize and to practice. Practically, this approach means that the same physician cares for each family member. This characteristic distinguishes family physicians from pediatricians and internists, who do not care for all family members because their patients are within specified age limits. Research using this conceptualization deals with family characteristics or events which can be summed such as family income, expenditure for medical services, number of illnesses or accidents, and number of physician visits or days of hospitalization per unit of time.

Individual in Family Context. This concept occurs with some frequency in other specialties and is the basic unit for the large body of research on psychosomatic disorders and their treatment of psychosomatic illness, and for psychotherapy and psychoanalysis. Only the individual patient may be seen by the physician, but the patient is encouraged to reveal family relationships which may be influencing his/her health. In these instances family is often viewed as contributing to the etiology of the presenting complaint.

Perhaps less prevalent is physicians' involvement of families in the long-term medical care and rehabilitation of patients with chronic diseases or physical disabilities. Many physicians have learned that families' involvement is important if patients are to carry out home care programs which require changes in diet, medication, therapeutic exercises, optimum rations of activity and rest, and use of prostheses. Although physicians' primary attention and concern are for the individual patient, members of the family are contacted by the physician to explain the details of the prescribed home care program and to enlist their help with the patient. Physicians in all fields of medicine have a growing awareness that social support systems, often families, serve to prevent illness, reduce complications, and enhance recovery (Medalie & Goldbourt, 1976; Nuckolls, 1976).

In each of the above cases physicians are sensitive to family influences on their patients, but they are assuming responsibility for the individual patient and not the family group. However, by placing the patient in family context, physicians may improve accuracy of diagnosis and enhance outcomes of treatment.

Family as a Biosocial System. This model of family, although the most difficult to conceptualize and to implement, offers promise for improving the quality of health care delivery. Conceptually, this model of family incorporates "a growing interest in generalizing the biological system model, in which all the parts and processes of an organism are viewed as interdependent among themselves and with the external environment, for a broader concept in which the patient is viewed as part of a social system that is intimately related to his physical as well as emotional well-being" (Bruce, 1973, p. 4). The model incorporates as well the "rediscovery of the human, social, and cultural aspects of health and illness" (Mauksch, 1976).

Concern with psychological and social phenomena had its advent with Freud and developed further when social scientists began to investigate medical phenomena. A shift in emphasis to these concerns occurred within the medical field itself during a period when medicine had reached a plateau in scientific advances. Medicine had essentially conquered infectious disease but had made no new breakthroughs in curing chronic illness. Physicians are now reaching beyond the biological in search of other approaches to treatment of illness. Family as a biosocial system fits into this context and appears to be an appropriate unit of care for family physicians.

One notable attempt to begin to conceptualize the family as a biosocial system is that of Mauksch (1974). In this approach the family is seen as being composed of two sets of components: unit members (individuals) and linking processes.

> There may be several individuals with identical patterns of blood pressure, circadian rhythms, intelligence quotients, assertiveness, body weight and other individual properties. These identical individuals cease to be identical when evaluated as members of their respective families with widely differing companions. The individual data emerge

> as interactive forces within the properties of these other members and thus differ in, in fact, meaning and behavior.... Similarly, social and cultural characteristics such as values, skills, and role performances which may adequately describe a person in his various social settings do not necessarily predict the intra-family processes (pp. 522-3).

A number of different linking processes occur within the family which cannot be explained from individual characteristics. These include not only psychological and social interdependencies but physiological ones as well, raising such questions as: "Are there differences in the response of human organisms to sharing a bed in close proximity during sleep? How do such differences, if they occur, affect the biological function of sleep, the relationship of the individuals and the nature of health of the participants?" (p. 523).

Mauksch's main thesis is that the pattern of individual properties and linking processes that characterizes a given family is unique and distinctive and that "this unit itself represents a health relevant commodity" which he calls the family's "health estate" (p. 524). The health estate is composed of interaction of a very complex set of forces including health behaviors, attitudes, values, knowledge, and social roles, including sex roles within the family, as well as the physical condition of the various members of the family over time.

This view of family and health, if accepted, has several important research implications. We know relatively little about the nature of these linking processes and their relationship to health. Thus, a vast new area of research is opened and if pursued will tend to be interdisciplinary in character as well as heavily influenced by the social sciences. Clearly such a synergistic view of the family has important clinical implications. It increases the amount and complexity of the data that must be evaluated. And, in addition, this model of the family as the unit of care raises some difficult ethical questions for clinical practice. We know that the family is sometimes an arena of intense interaction, enduring responsibility, and both positive and negative emotional expression among family members. To whom does the family physician owe principal loyalty within the new conception of the family as the unit of care? What uses would be made of the information acquired while attending one member of the family that have implications for the health of the others? The physician/patient relationship within medicine is both ethically and legally confidential. What then is appropriate physician behavior if family is the unit of care?

Summary. It is precarious to speculate if or how family physicians may go beyond a conception of family as a sum total of individuals in developing new styles of practice. Many family physicians appear to treat individuals in family context and are concerned with the influence of families on etiology of disease, health maintenance, and management of illness and disability, but the exact nature of this style of practice is not well documented. The concept of family as a biosocial system will require interdisciplinary investigation by medical practitioners and social scientists. Obviously this component of family physicians' role is the most ambiguous, least standardized, and least evident in practice. Sources of definitions of family as the unit of care derive from interdisciplinary efforts of physicians and social scientists. If family physicians and social scientists collaborating investigate families as biosocial systems and advance the concept both in theory and practice, it is likely that they can develop an expertise which clearly differentiates family medicine from other specialties and permits a unique contribution to scientific knowledge and to the practice of medicine.

Concluding Note

Manifest in the problems of simultaneously forming and performing their new role, family physicians face dilemmas of continually balancing attention between their mission of reform and their desire to establish a respected position in the field of medicine, of being a part of established medicine yet representing patients and serving as their advocates, of having to choose both among and within role components those values and behaviors which they find legitimate and which they think should receive priority, and of deciding which aspects of their role should receive attention for further definition and development. At present, family medicine is a field marked by ambiguities, thus uncomfortable for those requiring rigid guidelines but exciting and challenging for those interested in creating new styles of practice.

Within family medicine changes in styles of practice have been a quiet reform which may be more aptly characterized as proceeding on a level of person-to-person contact rather than through collective protests. In day-to-day interactions with patients, family physicians strive to provide continuing, comprehensive, humanized care for patients and families who have become disenchanted with and apprehensive about the overspecialized, bureaucratic, episodic care now offered. Although there have been formal actions to establish this specialty, family physicians still are attempting to gain a respected and influential position in medicine and medical education through interactions with deans, hospital administrators, and physicians in other specialties.

Family physicians form an alternate culture within established medicine which is contrary to medicine's emphasis on laboratory science, advanced technology, specialization, and research. A primary arena for value conflicts is the inpatient services of other specialties which provide training rotations for family medicine residents. These residents, who are being trained in one orientation to patient care by family physicians, enter the territory of other specialists with different orientations and criteria for performance. Similar types of conflicts in values occur when family physicians refer patients to other specialists. In outpatient family practice centers, family physicians functioning within their own territory are better able to implement their own approaches to patient care. In addition, to become and remain an approved family medicine residency requires that family practice centers meet certain specifications. These requirements provide leverage for negotiations with medical schools and hospitals for needed organizational changes, physical facilities, budget, and staff. Further sources of influence within medical schools in support of family medicine are state legislatures that have often budgeted funds and mandated the creation of family medicine departments or programs. Although it is yet too early to tell, it is likely that family medicine's greatest support will come from the public at large and the patients served. As family physicians continue to introduce reforms in patient care, they may gain further support from more and larger interest groups within the patient population.

Speculations about the future development of family physicians' role must be tentative. It appears likely that two role components–continuing, comprehensive care and humanized medicine– will receive considerable attention and will become institutionalized. The third component–family as the unit of care–is much more problematic, especially if family physicians choose to concentrate on treating families as biosocial systems. There are considerable difficulties, uncertainties, and problems involved; yet, development of this role component, if accomplished, promises a unique expertise for family physicians.

REFERENCE NOTES

1. My analysis is based on the following sources of information on family medicine: publications about the nature of the field which tend to be written by family physicians in academic positions and which for the most part are essays rather than empirical research; participant observation as a faculty member in a department of family medicine, attendance at professional meetings, and continuing dialogue with family physicians, residents, and medical students.

2. In the prevailing static approaches to the study of occupations, investigators tend to use functional analysis. Bucher and Strauss (1961) note that functionalists see a profession largely as a relatively homogeneous community whose members share identity, values, definitions of roles, and interests. Changes in the profession are viewed as deviations which are only temporal dislocations. Functional theory is inappropriate for

handling problems of development or change and seeks to explain present phenomenon in terms of its consequences for the continuity, persistence, stability, or survival of institutions (Buckley, 1967, p. 76). Thus, functional theory imposes inappropriate limitations for analysis of family medicine in its early stage of development.

3. For further reading on symbolic interaction, see for example: Blumer (1969); Lauer and Handel (1977); Manis and Meltzer (1967); Rose (1962); Schmitt (1972); and Shibutani (1961).

4. During the rise of specialization in medicine which has occurred in the last 50 years, general practitioners who had no residency training provided most of the primary care delivered in this country. Due to the lack of postdoctoral training, the medical establishment did not award these physicians the prestige conveyed to board certified specialists.

5. Stephens uses the term "patient management" to place emphasis on the interpersonal aspects of the family physicians' role in patient care in order to differentiate this component of the role from delivery of scientific medical care. "Management," however, is an unfortunate choice of terms for it connotes an authoritarian physician and a passive patient which is alien to family physicians' value system and is contrary to Stephens' intent.

6. Lynn (1977) notes that "the current role of family physician leads me to the assumption that the public demands three primary jobs of them: (1) they must provide first contact health care such that 85% to 95% of their illnesses will be handled without further referral; (2) they must provide expert referral to further health care resources in 5% to 15% of the cases; and (3) they must serve as health care and general counselor. Additionally, the public expects this health resource to be reasonably available within a short period of time from their home, school, place of work, or place of recreation. This role has been present in society in times past, and it appears to be a reasonable assumption that the demand for this role will continue. The current emphasis on family practice stemmed from a public perception that this role was not being well served, which resulted in political and economic forces being brought to bear to correct the situation."

7. See Stephens, 1976, for a discussion of social and cultural influences on the development of family medicine.

8. As one medical student pointed out, on a family practice rotation she did not feel the need to do a complete work-up during a single patient visit for she knew she would see the patient again. When she was based in the medicine outpatient clinic, she felt pressured to order extensive diagnostic tests because she might never see that patient again. Progressive rather than immediate use of intrusive approaches may depend heavily on physicians' expectations that contact with patients will be continuing.

9. The literature on psychosomatic medicine is extensive and easily accessible to the reader, thus references are not given here.

REFERENCES

Ad Hoc Committee on Education for Family Practice. *Meeting the challenge of family practice*. Chicago: American Medical Association (Willard Report), 1966.

American Academy of Family Physicians. Approved Family Practice Residencies. Chart. Kansas City: American Academy of Family Physicians, 1978.

Blau, R. et al. Cases and methods in humanistic medical care. Pp. 96-103 In S. Miller et al. (Eds.), *Dimensions of humanistic medicine*. San Francisco: The Institute for the Study of Humanistic Medicine, 1975.

Blumer, H. *Symbolic interactionism: Perspective and method.* Englewood Cliffs, NJ: Prentice-Hall, 1969.

Bruce, J. A. Family practice and the family: A sociological view. *Journal of Comparative Family Studies*, 1973, *4*(1), 4-12.
Bucher, R. Pathology: A study of social movements within a profession. *Social Problems*, 1962, *10*(1) 40-45.
Bucher, R., & Strauss, A. Professions in process. *American Journal of Sociology*, 1961, *66*, 325-334.
Buckley, W. *Sociology and modern systems theory*. Englewood Cliffs, NJ: Prentice-Hall, 1967.
Burke, K. *A grammar of motives*. New York: Prentice-Hall, 1945.
Carmichael, L. P. Teaching family medicine. *Journal of the American Medical Association*, 1965, *191*, 38-40.
Carmichael, L. P. Family medicine and practice. Letter to the editor. *Journal of the American Medical Association*, 1966, *198*, 953.
Carmichael, L. P. The family in medicine, process or entity. *Journal of Family Practice*, (1976) *3*(5), 521-525.
Carmichael, L. P. *Address to Society of Teachers of Family Medicine*. San Diego, CA, 1978.
Citizen's Commission on Graduate Medical Education. *The Graduate Education of Physicians*. Chicago: American Medical Association (Millis Report), 1966.
Cogswell, B. E. Variant family forms and life styles: Rejection of the traditional nuclear family. *The Family Coordinator*, 1975, *24*(4), 391-406.
Cogswell, B. E. Conceptual model of family as a group: family response to disability. In G. L. Albrecht (Ed.), *Socialization in the Disability Process*. Pittsburgh: University of Pittsburgh Press, 1976.
Cogswell, B. E., & Sussman, M. B. Changing families in changing environments: Implications for human service systems and population control. *Ohio Welfare Conference Bulletin*, 1972.
Cogswell, B. E., & Weir, D. D. A role in process: The development of medical professionals' role in long-term care of chronically diseased patients. *Journal of Health and Human Behavior*, 1964, *5*, 95-103.
Corea, G. *The hidden malpractice: How american medicine treats women as patients and professionals*. New York: William Morrow, 1977.
Curry, H. B. Strategy for achieving academic objectives of family medicine: Undergraduate education. Academic Missions of Family Medicine, *Fogarty International Center Proceedings Number 38*. United States Government Printing Office 017-044-00031-1, 1977.
Curtis, P., Rogers, J. The concept and measurement of continuity in primary care. *American Journal of Public Health*, 1980, *70*(2), 122-127.
Dubos, R. *Mirage of health; Utopias, progress and biological change*. New York: Harper, 1959.
Ehrenreich, B. & English, D. Complaints and disorders: The sexual politics of sickness. *Glass Mountain Pamphlet, Number 2*. Old Westbury, NY: The Feminist Press, 1973.
Flexner, A. Medical education in the United States and Canada. *A Report to the Carnegie Foundation for the Advancement of Teaching*. Bulletin of Medical Education, United States, Number Four, 1910.
Folsom, see National Commission on Community Health Services, 1966.
Frankfort, E. *Vaginal politics*. New York: Quadrangle Books, 1972.
Freidson, E. Profession of medicine–A study of the sociology of applied knowledge. New York: Harper and Row, 1970.
Geiger, H. J. The causes of dehumanization in health care and prospects for humanization. In J. Howard & A. Strauss (Eds.), *Humanizing health care*. New York: John Wiley and Sons, 1975.
Geyman, J. P., & Hawkes, G. R. A family-oriented perspective of behavioral science. The Syllabus for Teaching Behavioral Science in Family Practice. Acelomart, CA, 1973.

Gordis, L., & Markowitz, M. Evaluation of the effectiveness of comprehensive and continuous pediatric care. *Pediatrics*, 1971, *48*(5), 766-776.

Hill, R. Modern systems theory and the family: A confrontation. In M. B. Sussman (Ed.), *Sourcebook on marriage and the family*, (4th ed.). Boston: Houghton-Mifflin, 1974.

Howard, J. Humanization and dehumanization of health care: A conceptual view. In J. Howard & A. Strauss (Eds.), *Humanizing health care*. New York: John Wiley and Sons, 1975.

Howard, J., & Strauss, A., (Eds.). *Humanizing health care*. New York: John Wiley and Sons, 1975.

Illich, I. *Medical nemesis*. London: Marion Boyars, 1975.

Jason, H. Summary. *Academic Missions of Family Medicine, Fogarty International Center Proceedings Number 38*. United States Government Printing Office 017-044-00031-1, 1977.

Kennedy, E. *In critical condition: The crisis in american health care*. New York: Simon and Schuster, 1972.

Lauer, R. H., & Handel, W. H. *The theory and application of symbolic interactionism*. Boston: Houghton-Mifflin, 1977.

Litman, T. J. The family as a basic unit in health and medical care: A social-behavioral overview. *Social Science and Medicine*, 1974, *8*, 495-519.

Lynn, T. N. The future of family practice. *Continuing Education*, 1977, *2*, 24-25.

Manis, J. G., & Meltzer, B. N. (Eds.). *Symbolic interaction*. Boston: Allyn and Bacon, 1967.

Mauksch, H. O. A social science basis for conceptualizing family health. *Social Science and Medicine*, 1974, *8*, 521-528.

McWhinney, I. R. Continuity of care in family practice: Implications of continuity. *Journal of Family Practice*, 1975, *2*, 373-374.

Mechanic, D. Introduction. In J. Howard & A. Strauss (Eds.), *Humanizing health care*. New York: John Wiley and Sons, 1975.

Medalie, J. H., & Goldbourt, U. Angina pectoris among 10,000 men. *The American Journal of Medicine*, 1976, *60*(6), 910-921.

Miller, S. et al. *Dimensions of humanistic medicine*. San Francisco: The Institute for the Study of Humanistic Medicine, 1975.

Millis, J. See Citizens' Commission on Graduate Medical Education, 1966.

National Commission on Community Health Services. *Health is a community affair*. Cambridge, MA: Harvard University Press, (Folsom Report), 1966.

Nuckolls, K. B. Life crises and psychosocial assets: Some clinical implications. In B. H. Kaplan & J. C. Cassel (Eds.), *Family and health: An epidemiological approach*. Chapel Hill: Institute for Research in Social Science, 1975.

Olsen, E. H. The impact of serious illness on the family system. *Postgraduate Medicine*, 1970, *47*, 169-174.

Parsons, T. The sick role and the role of the physician reconsidered. *Milbank Memorial Fund Quarterly*, 1975, *53*, 257-278.

Pelligrino, E. D. The academic viability of family medicine: A triad of challenges. *Journal of the American Medical Association*, 1978, *240*, 132-135.

Phillips, T. J. Education and training of family physicians in the United States. Presented at Pan American Federation of Association of Medical Schools, New Orleans, LA, 1978.

Pisacano, N. J. The American board of family practice. In R. B. Taylor (Ed.), *Family medicine principles and practice*. New York: Springer-Verlag, 1978.

Pratt, L. *Family structure and effective health behavior: The energized family*. Boston: Houghton-Mifflin, 1976.

Ramey, J. Experimental family forms—the family of the future. *Marriage and Family Review*, 1978, *1*, 3-9.

Ransom, D., & Vandervoort, H. E. The development of family medicine: Problematic trends. *Journal of the American Medical Association*, 1973, *225*, 1098-1102.

Ransom, D. The Rise of Family Medicine: New Roles for Behavioral Science. (This issue) *Marriage and Family Review*.

Remen, N. et al. *The masculine principle, the feminine principle and humanistic medicine*. San Francisco: The Institute for the Study of Humanistic Medicine, 1975.

Rose, A. M. (Ed.). *Human behavior and social processes*. Boston: Houghton-Mifflin, 1962.

Schmitt, R. L. *The reference other orientation*. Carbondale, IL: Southern Illinois University Press, 1972.

Shibutani, T. *Society and personality*. Englewood Cliff, NJ: Prentice-Hall, 1961.

Smith, H. L. Psychiatry: A social institution in process. *Social Forces*, 1955, *33*(4).

Smith, H. L. Crisis in an institutional network: Community health care. In H. S. Becker, B. Geer, D. Roseman, R. S. Weiss (Eds.), *Institutions and the person: Papers presented to Everett C. Hughes*. Chicago: Aldine Publishing Company, 1968.

Somers, A. R. What price comprehensive care? *Archives of Environmental Health*, 1968, 17, 6-20.

Stephens, G. G. The intellectual basis of family practice. *The Journal of Family Practice*, 1975, *2*(6), 423-428.

Stephens, G. G. Reform in U.S.: Its impact on medicine and education for family practice. *Journal of Family Practice*, 1976, *3*, 507-512.

Strauss, A. L. *Mirrors and masks*. Glencoe, IL: The Free Press, 1959.

Strauss, A. L. A sociologist's perspective. In J. Howard & A. Strauss (Eds.), *Humanizing health care*. New York: John Wiley and Sons, 1975.

Szasz, T. S., & Hollender, M. H. The basic models of the doctor-patient relationship. *Archives of Internal Medicine*, 1956, *97*, 585-592.

Turner, R. Role taking: Process versus conformity. In A. M. Rose (Ed.), *Human behavior and social process: An interactionist approach*. Boston: Houghton-Mifflin, 1962.

Vincent, C. The family in health and illness: Some neglected areas. *Annals of the American Academy of Political and Social Science*, 1963, *346*, 109-115.

Waitzkin, H., & Waterman, B. *The exploitation of illness in capitalist society*. New York: Bobbs-Merrill, 1974.

Walsh, J. G. New specialty–family practice. *Journal of the American Medical Association*, 1970, *212*(7), 1191-1195.

Walton, R. F. Invited discussion. *Academic Missions of Family Medicine, Fogarty International Center Proceedings Number 38*. United States Government Printing Office 017-044-00031-1, 1977.

Willard, W. R. See Citizens' Commission on Graduate Medical Education, 1966.

Worby, C. M. The family life cycle: An orienting concept for the family practice specialist. *Journal of Medical Education*, 1971, *46*, 198-203.

THE RISE OF FAMILY MEDICINE: NEW ROLES FOR BEHAVIORAL SCIENCE

Donald C. Ransom, PhD

Introduction

The aim of this paper is to approach the field of family medicine as a clinical behavior scientist.* In doing so I will provide an orientation to the meaning, content, and applications of family medicine together with a discussion of some issues raised by taking the family approach in clinical settings. It is not my intent to define the field in a fixed way. Quite the contrary, any definitions or assertions should be taken only for their heuristic value.

Family Medicine

In two earlier papers, Vandervoort and I (Ransom & Vandervoort, 1973; Vandervoort & Ransom, 1973) provided a general conception of family medicine, emphasizing the importance of introducing the study of human relatedness and health in medical education and suggesting that the greatest promise of the new specialty of family practice lay in focusing on primary groups as both subjects and objects of health care.

The dual concerns of understanding and changing originally described in these papers seem clear enough today. Family medicine is both a field of

---

Dr. Ransom is Associate Professor in Residence, Division of Family and Community Medicine, University of California School of Medicine, San Francisco, CA 94143, and Behavioral Science Coordinator, Family Practice Residency Program, Community Hospital of Sonoma County, 3325 Chanate Rd., Santa Rosa, CA 95402.

The author wishes to express his gratitude to Elaine Bauserman, William Gerber, Betty Cogswell, and Bruce Denner, who read an earlier draft of this paper and provided valuable comments and corrections that were incorporated into the present version.

---

*Throughout this paper, the categorical noun, "behavioral science" or "the behavioral sciences" (no specific distinction is implied by the use of either the singular or plural term), is meant to be applied in the broadest possible sense that still allows the designation to be meaningful. Thus, I mean to employ the first of two major definitions discussed by Badgley and Bloom, "a comprehensive view including an array of biological, psychological, and social sciences in collaborative inquiry concerning human behavior" (1973, p. 928), following especially in the systems–transdisciplinary tradition of James E. Miller (1955), Anthony Wilden (1972), and Gregory Bateson (1972).

Marriage & Family Review, Vol. 4(1/2), Spring/Summer 1981

inquiry and an applied discipline with neither territory fenced in by a single professional specialty. What seemed clear at the time of the earlier presentation but, apparently, becomes obscured when the term *family* is used repeatedly as the noun and adjective of choice, is that it is not the family as entity or institution that is of central concern, but "family" as a metaphoric designation for primary, largely self-regulated human systems. Thus, family medicine is concerned with any group that makes a significant difference in its members' lives. More important than paying attention to any particular corporate group is "family mindedness" among providers, as health problems are conceptualized, defined, and addressed in relation to their specific contexts.* Thus, family medicine is concerned with the formal as well as the concrete and personal aspects of human relatedness and health.

Background

Looking back, it appears that attention to the family and health has been cyclical. Each renewal of interest has failed to generate sufficient momentum to launch family issues and concerns into the mainstream of medicine. We are now witnessing a new high point on a cyclical curve which last peaked just before the United States entered in World War II.

Spiegel and Bell (1959) have outlined the historical background of interest in the family shown by psychiatry, social work, and sociology since the late nineteenth century. No such chronicle has been written about general medical interest in the family, though Alpert and Charney (1973) provide a brief history of efforts to expose medical students to families. A history of family medicine remains to be written. Only a few of the most significant developments contributing to the present day shape of the field will be mentioned here.

The modern history of family-centered care begins with the "Peckham Experiment" (Pearse & Williamson, 1931; Williamson & Pearse, 1939; Pearse & Crocker, 1943). In 1926, a "family club" was opened in a small house in the Southeast London borough of Camberwell. It was equipped with a consulting room, receptionist's office, bath and changing room, and one small club room. By the end of 3 years 112 families had joined and all the members of those families had presented themselves for a "periodic health overhaul." In 1935, a three-story, 58,000 square feet structure, the "Pioneer Health

*Sluzki (1974) discusses the importance of the transformation from lineal, dichotomous thinking to "thinking interactionally" or "thinking family" that occurs when family practice residents encounter ideological and institutional support for a contextual–ecological epistemology.

Centre," was built. "It was a great venture; a social structure to be built with a new unit—not the individual but *the family*" (Pearse & Crocker, 1943, p. 13). The Centre contained a small health clinic including a laboratory. In addition, it housed a large swimming pool, gymnasium, game rooms, a music room, library and quiet room, work rooms, nursery, a large dance floor with stage, a theater, a self-service cafeteria and pub, a store, outdoor grounds, and eventually the operation expanded to incorporate a summer camp and a cooperative farm seven miles away. At its peak, enrollment reached about 1,400 families, all living in the principally lower-middle and middle class neighborhood, within a mile ("walking distance") of the Centre.

In the beginning, the aim was to construct a setting "designed to be furnished with people and their actions" (Pearse & Crocker, 1943, p. 69). It was a "biologist's" living laboratory. The purpose was to study life *in vivo* and thereby study health rather than illness. The staff remained constant and small. In the end, brought on by the War in 1939, it was clear to those involved that the best way to improve individual health was to strengthen the family through providing opportunities for growth and self-care within the wider social and physical environment.

The Pioneer Health Care Centre was not a "polyclinic" of the type familiar in those days and it did not provide comprehensive "sickness care" services. Its main functions were social. Medically, its important service was to provide annual combined physical examinations and consultations called the "family health overhaul" in which the results and implications were discussed with the family as a group. The policy was "information without advice," although advice was freely given.

A variety of health related activities were sponsored by the Centre, including prenatal counseling for couples, swimming and exercise classes for pregnant women, the sale of fresh raw milk and organic vegetables, and the detection of a surprising degree of previously undiagnosed disorders. In addition the Centre sponsored an alternative birth arrangement with a nearby teaching hospital whereby "mothers could be received for the period of 48 hours covering the delivery, after which they returned home with their babies" in contrast with the 2-week period of "confinement" customary at the time.

The Centre's commitment to health through human development in the broadest sense is exemplified by an experiment begun in the summer of 1939 and cut short by the War, in which Maria Montessori laid the plans for an educational nursery for children aged 1 1/2 years and upwards, including their mothers. The purpose in involving mothers was "so that in helping with the education of their own children not only might they come through practice to understand the essence of education, but that they might also simultaneously renew their own education long since forgotten and foregone"(Pearse & Crocker, 1943, p. 317).

Four years after the Pioneer Health Centre was built, the Josiah Macy, Jr. Foundation funded "The Study of the Family in Sickness and Health Care." Shepherded by Lawrence K. Frank of the Macy Foundation and infused with his ideas (e.g., see *Society as the Patient*, 1949, a collection of Frank's essays), the study was a cooperative venture among members of the faculties of public health, medicine, and psychiatry at Cornell University Medical College, and included representatives from social work and nursing from New York Hospital. A group of 15 families was studied over a 2-year period with the goals of understanding "the interrelation between illness and the family situation," learning something about the "implications for treatment" following from such an approach, and then "exploring the best methods for cooperative treatment" with the family health care team assembled for the study (Richardson, 1945, pp. 312-313). The report of that study, *Patients Have Families*, was prepared by Henry B. Richardson, the project's director.

What the Peckham Experiment provided in commitment to total health and dedication to establishing the family as "the unit of living," the Macy Family Study matched with a formal description of the family as a system that operates to influence the health and illness of its members and to regulate their access to health care and community resources. Published by the Commonwealth Fund in 1945, *Patients Have Families** is an early example of the contribution the social and behavioral scientist's imagination can make to the conceptualization and study of health and disease. Margaret Mead was a member of the study group and was responsible for designing the research and later organizing the family case studies and team conference notes for the book. In addition, the basic conceptual framework was provided by Mead, based on her own work, (e.g., "The Concept of Culture and the Psychosomatic Approach" written in 1940 but not published until 1947). Thus, it is not surprising to find such statements in the book as, "the doctor who treats the patient for a chronic disease may be observing one aspect of a reciprocating system of which he may become aware if he inquires into the health of the family" (p. 324). The presentation in *Patients Have Families* anticipated Don Jackson's (1957) notion of "family homeostasis" by 15 years. In chapters entitled, "The Family Equilibrium" and "Different Types of Family Equilibrium," and in general in an appendix called "Concepts Relative to the

*Although the book went through four printings, the last in 1948, it is now virtually lost to modern students of the family and health, having no Library of Congress Card Catalog number and being long since out of print.

Family Equilibrium," the general idea is spelled out and six mechanisms that serve to maintain the "family equilibrium" are described.

Richardson and his Family Study team appear now to have been working with a vision of American medicine that was 30 years ahead of its time. In the final paragraph of the introduction to *Patients Have Families* they say, "In summary, the profession of medicine progressed from the diseased organ to the total personality of the patient, and is now ready for the concept of the individual as a member of a family in its community setting" (p. xviii). Perhaps they were taken by the excitement of interdisciplinary work or the promise of new ideas from cybernetics, a field whose early development was supported by a series of conferences sponsored by the same people within the Macy Foundation who were supporting their work. Perhaps Richardson's own clinical experiences had convinced him that family-centered medicine was the next logical step. In any case, the War intervened, and when it was over, the next 20 years were to witness the greatest investment in biomedical technological research and emphasis on subspecialization in the history of medicine. Family medicine remained in the chrysalis.

As "The Study of Family in Sickness and Health Care" was drawing to a close, a related project was being planned. Inspired by the Peckham Experiment, Baily B. Burritt persuaded the Community Service Society and the Milbank Memorial Fund to support what eventually became "The Family Health Maintenance Demonstration" of the Montefiore Medical Group, a comprehensive health care option of the Health Insurance Plan of Greater New York. Located at Montefiore Hospital and affiliated with the Columbia University College of Physicans and Surgeons, the Demonstration was in the planning stages from 1943 to 1950 and then ran for 9 years under the direction of George A. Silver, MD.

Like Richardson's Family Study, the Family Health Maintenance Demonstration combined research with service. Over a 5-year period a wide range of data were collected on 100 families matched against a roughly equal number of controls and then compared. Study families were provided with a team consisting of an internist, a pediatrician, a public health nurse, and a social worker, and all available specialty and ancillary services as needed. The centrality of the family and the importance of disease prevention were values to be stressed. The results of the individuals enrolled were in general favorable, but as an experiment in providing health services the Demonstration left us with more information about what not to do then how to put the family approach into practice.

In *Family Medical Care: A Report on the Family Health Maintenance Demonstration*, Silver (1963) describes a number of reasons why the Demonstration struggled, including the difficulties of team coordination and the reluctance of professionals to try out new roles.* But what is most striking in retrospect is that the group involved did not draw upon conceptual models of the family close at hand to guide them in their organization of services, interventions, and research. The psychological and interpersonal dimension of their work was dominated instead by an individual intrapsychic orientation.

The "family-as-organism" model of the Peckham Experiment did not influence the study. Another curious fact is that the work of the Macy Family Study team is not mentioned in Silver's report, an anomaly since both groups worked in New York, since Baily B. Burritt, the original guiding force of the Demonstration, was also on the "Technical Committee" that oversaw the Macy Family Study, and since the nascent systems model developed in *Patients Have Families* could have been of enormous benefit to the Family Health Maintenance Demonstration's purposes. These omissions seem all the more tragic in the light of one of the most revealing statements in Silver's book, that the routine family health conference, modeled after the "family health overhaul" of the Peckham Experiment, "was perhaps the single most useful device employed by the Demonstration" (Silver, 1963, p. 199).

In the years since the publication of *Patients Have Families*, the major conceptual developments and practical methods for working with families have continued to come from the behavioral sciences, especially from the diverse group of psychologists, social workers, sociologists, anthropologists, and psychiatrists interested in family process and psychological disturbances, and family therapy. The early work of Bowen and his colleagues at the National Institute of Mental Health (e.g., Bowen et al., 1957) included having whole families with a schizophrenic member live on the ward together for up to six months, a dramatic move toward focusing on the family as the unit of analysis and approaching the family as the patient. The work of Wynne (e.g., Wynne et al., 1958), and later Wynne and Singer, following Bowen at NIMH; Lidz and his co-workers at Yale (e.g., Lidz, Fleck, & Cornelison, 1965); and the Bateson Group in Palo Alto all supplied important grounding concepts and established a language for thinking about families that was rooted in terms of communication and group process rather than energy and personality dynamics.

One of the Palo Alto group, Don Jackson, eventually published two papers on family practice (1965, 1966), emphasizing the general systems approach and calling attention to the way medical problems affect and are affected by

*See also *Family Medical Care: A Design for Health Maintenance*, George A. Silver (1974), a revision and extension of the earlier work.

the "family homeostasis." Important recent extensions of this tradition that are directly related to family medicine include the research of Minuchin and his colleagues in Philadelphia (e.g., Minuchin et al., 1975 and 1978, discussed here p. 18-20) on the family and psychosomatic disease; the investigation of "family somatics" by Weakland (1977), Hoebel (1977), and associates in Palo Alto; and the work of Sluzki (1974, 1976) in San Fransisco, Bauman and Grace (1974) in Santa Rosa, California, Geyman (1978) in Seattle, and Medalie (1978) in Cleveland, directly in family practice residency training and family health care.

Contributions to the development of family medicine have also come from pediatrics, traditional general practice, medical social work, medical sociology and anthropology, rehabilitation specialties (especially those involved in home health care programs), and numerous other groups and individuals who have worked in relative isolation and with little support. A variety of these will be noted in the next section. Overall, family health research projects and family health programs have had a difficult time in the face of indifference or opposition from predominantly biomedically minded subspecialists who generally control funds and space. Few survived, until the establishment of family practice as a medical specialty in 1969.

The contributions of general practice in England are consistently helpful (e.g., Kellner, 1963; Clyne, 1961), but over the years have had little impact on either American family practice or family medicine. While the British do a great deal of practical work as family physicians, there appears to be no special emphasis on the family as an emergent system. There is no prevalent conceptual model of the family in evidence in the British literature beyond that of a group of interacting personalities. British medical and social science has always had a difficult time with the proposition that a group of persons can be viewed as a general system and as such described with terms such as "healthy" and "pathological" that ordinarily apply only to individuals (e.g., Laing & Esterson, 1964; McEwan, 1974; Black, 1976; Marinker, 1976).*

The importance of societal influences on the development of family medicine should not be underestimated. These include mass media, changing patterns of government funding and the development of a national health policy, the maldistribution of physicans and the shortage of primary care services, the changing emphasis from "sickness cure" to "health care," and changing attitudes toward health providers exemplified in the consumer movement and the women's movement. They are simply too extensive and complex to summarize here.

The decisive breakthrough for family medicine occurred in 1969 when

*A full discussion of the family as a system can be found in Ransom and Massad (1978).

"family practice" was officially recognized by the American Medical Association as the 20th specialty in American medicine. The American Board of Family Practice was established and resident training was systematically undertaken. Family practice was to provide a well-trained personal physician who would offer comprehensive, continuing care to all age groups, accepting the responsibility for providing or coordinating patients' total health care needs in their revelant social contexts. A large gap in the health care system was on the way to being closed. Even more important for the vitality of family medicine as an emerging discipline than the establishment of the specialty, however, was the insistence by the Committee on Education of the American Board of Family Practice that each residency program create a "model family practice unit," separate and distinct from other ambulatory care services and "unique to family practice." Approval would not be granted without such a structure. Thus, a special place to work was provided, not just for family practice residents, but for the wide variety of personnel who shared a common interest in families and health who had previously carried on without a common rallying ground and base of operations.

Research

From the standpoint of family medicine as a field of inquiry, it is important to establish a frame of reference bounding its major concerns and distinguishing its efforts from either predominantly individual approaches (intraperson, single-organism variables) or larger community and societal approaches (political and economic variables, social policy and public health). A "middle range" of variables invites opportunities to study familial, work group, and immediate social environmental contexts in relation to health, illness, and care, and provides a focal point for research.

The potential for research in family medicine has only begun to be realized. However, enough provocative work has been done to recognize that a body of knowledge exists and a field of expertise is in the making. Contributions have come from all the major disciplines within the social and behavioral sciences and from several disciplines within the medical and nursing specialties. Investigations fall naturally into groups of studies with common concerns. It is useful to delineate four overlapping categories, which, for the present, can serve as an outline of the dimensions or content of family medicine*:

1. Family roles in the etiology, mediation, and maintenance of illness.

*These categories are limited to studies of family processes proper. Research on the design and delivery of health services, studies of the education of eventual providers, and other questions of importance to the total field of family medicine are not included here.

2. Effects on the family and its members of illness and the treatment of illness.
3. Family-health services provider relations.
4. The family as its own health restoring and health promoting agency.

These dimensions are surveyed below. No effort is made to review the literature; it is simply too large to handle here. Studies are cited simply to illustrate the contents and boundaries of family medicine as it is defined here.**

1. Family Roles in Illness

From the beginning of the life cycle to the end, families affect the health of their members in virtually every conceivable way. We quickly think of genetic transmission leading to hereditary diseases or relative strengths; food, clothing, shelter, and the differences resulting from their infinite varieties; the transmission of health habits and values leading to biological and emotional strengths and vulnerabilities; differences in the perception and tolerance of sickness and norms governing the sick role; and events in the family leading to differential effects on members. Social interaction in families affects health in more subtle ways then these, and the understanding of such relationships has only begun to be studied systematically.

There is abundant evidence that the health of young children is largely determined by the family environment, although the mediation of such influence is open to a wide variety of debatable, alternative interpretations. The classic study of families in Newcastle upon Tyne, England (Miller et al., 1960), found that mortality in the first year of life was four times greater among children born out of marriage than within. The families studied were rated in terms of group variables signifying deprivation, deficiency, and dependency. For the 53% of families described as having at least one of these system conditions (out of 847 families observed for 5 years) there was found a significantly higher incidence of staphylococcal disease, tuberculosis, gastrointestinal disease, reduced height, enuresis, and convulsions compared to the group who were free of the conditions of deprivation, deficiency and dependency.

**My focus here is on questions involving the family and health and illness that fall outside the traditional concerns of the family and mental health and illness, mental retardation, and learning disorders. This literature is enormous and is well-known and no purpose is served by attempting to encompass it here. By no means do I wish to suggest a dichotomy between physical health and mental health and questions of learning. Nor do I wish to suggest that these issues fall outside the scope of family medicine. Quite the contrary, they are incorporated within all the dimensions outlined above.

Lack of parental interaction and support has consistently been found to be crippling to the development of young children. Spitz's (1945, 1947) widely quoted study of foundling homes versus nursery care related maternal and social deprivation to increased infant mortality, susceptibility to disease, retardation in growth, and failure to achieve developmental milestones. Whereas the Spitz study compared the effects of interaction between two highly specialized environments, McCarthy and Booth (1970) found evidence of a syndrome resembling Spitz' "hospitalism" occurring in children living at home with their parents. The most prominent abnormalities they described were dwarfism and subnormal weight/height ratios, interestingly, with little or no evidence of malnutrition. Behaviorally, the children exhibited varying degrees of bodily neglect, apathy, subnormal intelligence, and the inability to play.

When these children from 10 families were removed from their homes and placed in the hospital, where it is assumed that a different type of interaction occurred between them and the staff than occurred in their homes, their symptoms, including the dwarfism, were reversed in most cases. While this study was focused explicitly on mothers, like so many studies of mother-infant interaction, the kind of relationship that developed could not have been made possible without either the absence of a father or other available caregiver(s). Behind many studies of negative dyadic interactions is a larger family drama. Such patterns are significantly more difficult to conceptualize and to investigate than the study of dyads.

At the opposite end of the life cycle, a study by Greene, Goldstein, and Moss (1972) of the psychosocial aspects of sudden death found that among men who developed myocardial infarction, considerable psychological distress had been evoked by circumstances in which there were departures or current disappointing conflicts between the patient and son or daughter, especially a son.

Van Heijingen (1966) noted a similar pattern when he reported that rejection by a loved one frequently preceded the clinical emergence of coronary disease.

Loss of social supports–particularly loss of a spouse–has been implicated over and over again in rapidly deteriorating health and, not uncommonly, death. Studies of psychosocial correlates of the onset of cancer repeatedly point to torn family relationships as high risk factors in the development of cancer. Similarly, when Parkes, Benjamin, and Fitzgerald (1969) followed the death rates of 4,486 widowers of 55 years of age and older for 9 years following the death of their wives, they found that 213 died during the first 6 months of bereavement, 40% over the expected death rate for married men of the same ages. The death rate from degenerative heart disease was 67% above what would be expected. If the widowers survived the first year beyond the death of their wives their mortality rate dropped to that of married men. Kiritz and Moos (1974) provide an excellent review of a wide range of research that correlates relationship dimensions such as support, cohesion, and involvement with physiological changes.

Psychosomatic medicine has recently begun to expand its interest to infectious dieases. Friedman and Glasgow (1966) point out that psychogenic diseases are typically thought of as those in which either psychological factors directly cause a pathological state, or characterological factors predispose a person to specific syndromes. In the first instance, a given emotional crisis or series of psychological upheavals might be sought for in a patient whose symptoms could not be explained on an "organic" basis. In the second instance, where characterological elements are suspected a person might be designated as a "peptic ulcer type." Clinical studies continue to suggest that such formulations contain some elements of truth and lead us to revise and extend our scope to include family patterns and family types as predisposing factors.

Psychosomatics has been joined by "family somatics" (Weakland, 1977) as personality systems now share the focus of investigation with small social systems. With this expansion into complex levels of interaction, persons with infections and "organic" diseases of all kinds are now as interesting to psychosomatic and family somatic inverstigators as persons with what traditionally have been called psychosomatic illnesses.

Since infectious disease is a product of a special type of relation, we are now beginning to study the interaction of co-respondents in that relation. This has meant shifting the focus of attention from the microorganism in the laboratory to the study of the host in the natural environment. Defining the unit to be called "host" is itself an interesting problem. Though conventionally host status is assigned to an individual, it can also be useful to think of the family as host, though one of its members may be in more active relation with an "uninvited guest" than the others at a given moment. One of the major contributions of family medicine generally is that it continually raises the question, "which units–of observation, analysis, assessment, intervention–shall we employ?"

Growing interest in these kinds of questions has led investigators into the "interior" of the family to explore the ways in which family organization and behavior may constitute immunological structures and thereby affect the immunological competence of individual members. Meyer and Haggerty (1962) looked directly at the influence of family crises upon resistance to infection. Studying a group of families in the Family Medicine Unit at Boston Children's Hospital, they found that common crises, such as the death of a grandparent, a change of residence, loss of father's job, and a child's being subjected to unusual pressure, occurs four times more frequently in the 2-week period prior to the appearance of streptococcal infections than in the two weeks afterward. Many other family factors were also found to influence susceptibility to illness. The general pattern of their findings are consistent with those of Mutter and Shleifer (1966), and Schmale (1958) and Schottstaedt, et al., (1958).

The common crises uncovered by Meyer and Haggerty are virtually identical with a number of "life event items" in Holmes and Rahe's widely cited Social Readjustment Rating Scale (SRRS). Holmes and Rahe found that events constituting significant change, wanted or unwanted, pleasant or unpleasant, increase a person's vulnerability to all sorts of illnesses and accidents. Studying several populations, they found a consistent relationship between the magnitude of life changes and the timing and seriousness of the illness experienced. Of special interest here is that of the top 40 life event items in the SRRS (weighted according to their adaptive requirements); 26 are directly "intrafamilial" and eight more constitute work or financial changes that very likely would also directly affect a family's life.

The general notion of "stress" is the most obvious and widely cited factor linking families and individual susceptibility, but in its general usage, the meaning of stress is too undifferentiated to be of much clinical use. Recent conceptualizations are more specific and also more complex (e.g., Lazarus, 1977). Moss (1973) reviewed interactionally relevent conceptualizations of stress and suggested a set of relations between social participation, physiological processes, and disease susceptibility. His conceptualization of stress is defined partly in cognitive terms and is concerned with informational incongruities and group's ability to protect its members from them. Work of this kind is paving the way toward an understanding of relations between meaning and immunity at the social as well as the cellular level.

Among the most complex problems yet studied are family factors involved in the onset and course of autoimmune diseases. In family medicine this problem is viewed as an aspect of the general question concerning how relationships with others affect one's relationship to oneself. The results from biological research demonstrate that the genetic system's "predisposition" to develop into a particular biological structure can be significantly altered by encountering a novel environment. Suspending temporarily the idea that genetic instructions and biological structures are "hard" compared to social instructions and biosocial structures which are "soft," it is not unreasonable to think that persons interacting with their family environments in unique ways will undergo changes that may be adaptive at one level of organization but problematic at another. McClary, Meyer, and Weitzman (1955), and Otto and Mackay (1967) found that onset lupus erythematosis frequently followed major life stress situations. Solomon and Moos (e.g., 1965b) found interesting differences between siblings stemming from early childhood experiences, in which different roles were assumed in the family. These role differences correlate with active rheumatoid arthritis in adult life, even when controlled for the presence of rheumatoid factor in the paired siblings' blood.

Turning to another kind of problem, family roles are central when one looks closely at the natural history of accidents. Accidents are the leading cause of death and disability in children after the newborn period. Meyer et al. (unpublished, cited by Haggerty & Alpert, 1963) compared the families of 113 preschool children who were involved in accidents serious enough to require hospitalization with the families of 103 children who were not involved in accidents. Of many interesting connections linking family events and accidents, their most concrete and dramatic finding was that 54% of the accidents they followed occurred at a time when an immediate family member, especially the mother, was ill.

In addition to the etiological roles we have been considering, families mediate the course of illness in a variety of ways. The failure to call for help until it is too late was documented in several cases in the accident study. In less direct ways the meaning an illness may hold for a family collectively can determine responses to it. Occasionally the threat of an illness is so great that a "stimulus-barrier" performs the specific function of excluding or greatly inhibiting assimilation of information into the family system (Shands, 1951, 1966, 1970). Thus, the failure to recognize symptoms, seek medical opinion, or "accept" diagnostic information or medical advice may involve active avoidance or denial, a problematic response in relation to the potential benefits of some current therapies, the success of which depends on early recognition and treatment.

Research in family medicine has taken a recent developmental leap with the work of Minuchin and his colleagues at the Philadelphia Child Guidance Clinic and the Children's Hospital of Philadelphia (e.g., Minuchin, 1974; Minuchin et al., 1975; Minuchin, Rosman, & Baker, 1978). The Minuchin group has provided the first major extension of the systems approach to the study of the family and psychosomatic illness since the work of Jackson and Yalom (1955). Their work is opening the way for the first potentially important advances, both in theory and practice, since the series of contributions by Alpert, Charney, Haggerty, Kosa, Meyer, and Roghmann and their co-workers in Boston and Rochester during the 1960s.

Let us briefly assess this recent work in its historical context. Most previous work in the area designated by the term family medicine, including most of the studies referred to in this discussion, has suffered from two major problems. First it has been bound by a prevailing conceptual language that decribes and explains human health behavior in lineal terms. Situation-personality-emotion-physiological change-bodily distress are linked in series in a causal chain. To the extent that such a language allows for conceptualizations of interactions, they are usually of the "billiard ball" type. A family environment surrounds and is therefore seen as relevant to understanding the behavior of its members in the same way that a billiard table contains balls (imposing constraints, for example) with members affecting one another through their contact the way balls impact upon and react to one another on the table. Illness is seen as a property of the individual, a product of interacting with his or her environment, the way an imperfectly rolling billiard ball might be described as worn down as a result of bumping too intensely and too often against its neighboors, rather than viewed as a property of the group acting as a unit. In short, when family members are described as "collaterals" instead of members of a mutually bounded system, the ecological metaphor capable of advancing our conceptualization of an individual's state of health to that of a product of interaction between systems or between levels within a system is not possible.

The second problem is that most research investigating family behavior and health has not been linked to health care delivery and, as a result, theory, research, and practice have benefited very little from one another over the years.

The Philadelphia group is addressing both of these problems directly. In the first case they are extending and refining an open-linked systems model which redefines certain psychosomatic processes by describing them as disorders of the group as well as disorders of the individual. In their study of psychosomatic illness in children this shift is facilitated by two postulates: "(1) that certain types of family organization are closely related to the development and maintenance of psychosomatic symptoms in children, and (2) that children's psychosomatic symptoms play a major role in maintaining family homeostasis" (Minuchin et al., 1975, p. 1032). Examples of family patterns associated with psychosomatic illness are "enmeshment," "overprotectiveness," "rigidity," and "lack of conflict resolution." The sick child's role in the family's pattern of conflict avoidance is an important source of reinforcement for his symptoms. When these conditions are combined with an additional postulate of physiological vulnerability, a useful multilevel systems model is made available for research and intervention.

In the second case, the construction of this conceptual model has gone hand in hand with the treatment of psychosomatogenic families. The team involved in research is also involved in therapy, and the success of both activities affirms the utility of this combination.

2. *Effects on the Family of Illness and Treatment*

Research problems in this category typically turn around the questions posed from the vantage point taken in studies outlined above. The family and family members' responses become dependent variables, as investigators search for ways in which illness and treatment lead to further disruption. adaptive responses, and reorganization.

Like the study of family roles in illness, the effects on the family of encountering illness and health services have been widely investigated by diverse groups within the health and behavioral sciences. Research reports frequently take the form, "The Impact on the Family of __________," with a broad range of illness and contacts with the health care system filling in the blank. Mental illness and the mental-hospitalization of a family member have received considerable attention, as have mental developmental abnormalities. Among illnesses traditionally described as "organic" or "physical," whole books and collections have been devoted to specific problems: e.g., Katz (1970) on hemophilia; Easson (1970) on the dying child; and Debuskey (1970) on the chronically ill child and his family—to sample just 1 year. Certain problems seem to command special attention, for instance, cystic fibrosis, (e.g., Meyerowitz & Kaplan, 1967; Anderson, 1960; Turk, 1964; Sojit, 1971), while others go unstudied.

Most research falling into the "impact on" group is generally concerned with families' reactions to and/or family members' attitudes about the illness or hospitalization of a member. Sometimes studies focus on the positive side, describing the adaptation process in terms of the mobilization of family resources, reallocation of role responsibilities, involvement of extended family members, cognitive restructuring, and the stages and phases of the "coping" process. Other studies focus more on the negative side, exploring the disrupting and destructive aspects of encountering illness and the health care system on family organization, resources, and solidarity, and on other individual members' health. A sample of investigations interested in the adaptation or coping process at the family level includes Ellenberger, Sangier, and Wittkower (1964), and Gordon and Kutner (1965) on the long-term and fatal illness of a child; Debuskey and contributors (1970) on 10 different chronic diseases of childhood; Kanoff, Kunter, and Gordon (1962) on the impact of genetic disease (Tay-Sachs); Meadows (1968) on congenital deafness; Lowenfeld (1964) on blind children; Davis (1963) on polio; Roghmann, Hecht, and Haggerty (1973) on acute illness of children; Chodoff, Friedman, and Hamburg (1963) on children with malignant disease; Jacobson and Eichhorn (1964) on heart disease; Sussman (1953, 1959) on patterns of helping during illness; and Sussman and Slater (1963) on the rehabilitation process.

A sample of studies concerned with the ways in which illness in a member can lead to additional problems for the family includes Vaughn (1968) on the effect on families of experiencing sudden infant death; Maxwell and Gane (1962) on disorganizing anxiety in families with congenital heart disease; D'Arcy (1969) on the impact of congenital defects; Krush, Krush, and Lynch (1965) on community hostility and rejection projected on a family with a disfiguring genetic fault; Cook (1963) on family limitations following the birth of a cerebral palsied child; Crain, et al., (1966) on effects on marital integration of a diabetic child; Martin, Lawrie, and Wilkinson (1968) on enduring disturbances in families with a fatally burned child; Skipper et al. (1968) on problems in the marital relationship stemming from physical disability among women; Honegman et al. (1968) on the impact of heart disease; and Castro de la Mata, Gingras, and Wittkower (1960) on the impact of sudden, severe disablement of the father upon the family.

Specific consequences of efforts to cope with health crises have also been investigated. In one study, Friedman, Mason, and Hamburg (1963) found that adrenocortical functioning appears to be related to the effectiveness of coping and that the breakdown of efforts to manage a family crisis is associated with elevated corticosteriod levels. In a group of parents of children with leukemia, higher 18-hydroxycorticosteroid excretion rates were observed in those parents judged to be relatively ineffective in coping with the problems of caring for a fatally ill child.

In a major investigation of health care and the family over three generations, Litman (1971, 1974b) looked closely at the impact of illness on family solidarity. His data allowed him to observe the differential impact of acute versus chronic illness and to compare generational responses to what appear to be the same sorts of problems on the surface. He found that while most illnesses (75%) reportedly had little effect on family solidarity, of the remaining quarter, an equal number appeared either to have brought the family closer together or to have made relationships in the family more difficult. Summarizing his own work in the most extensive review available on the subject of "the family as a basic unit in health and medical care," Litman

(1974a) calls attention to interesting generational differences, with illness in the parent generation tending to have a more integrating effect and illness among their married children tending to have the opposite effect, increasing tension and anxiety. Discovering that families whose members were considered to be seriously ill were about as likely to have been brought together as driven apart, Litman pursued the subtleties of distinguishing between attitudes and/or preceptions and actual family relations. On the whole, he found that

> there appeared to be little, if any, evidence that perceived family solidarity, marital happiness or close family ties provides any particular hedge against the disruptive impact of a member's illness on family relations. As a matter of fact, if anything, the opposite appeared to be true. Whereas the cohesion of an extremely close, well-integrated and maritally happy family may be severely strained as a result of a member's illness, such an event may serve to bring those with more disparate family ties together. Why this should be so remains unclear and in need of further study (1974a, p. 509).

There are good theoretical reasons to expect that a family's response to illness would exemplify its customary pattern of responding to other types of stress. Cohen (1962) found evidence of this pattern in his study of family behavior surrounding a handicapped child. On the other hand, Litman (1974b) found that the ways and the extent to which a member's illness affected his or her family appeared to be a function of the nature of the illness itself. Expectably, the more prolonged and complicated the illness, the greater the likelihood it will lead to differences in family relatedness. Thus, while almost 60% of the acute cases studied by Litman reported little or no appreciable impact on family patterns, the reverse was true for those cases which were of a more chronic or complex nature.

We can begin to see that understanding family patterns of response to illness will require data and analytic models of greater complexity than past studies have provided. In future studies it would be helpful to know something about family members' cognitive styles, about families' patterns of organization, decision making, allocation of role behaviors, capacity to process novelty, articulation with extended family and community resources, and about relations with the health care system, including "third parties" involved in the financial picture, together with a clear picture of the type of illness confronting a family and the conventional pattern of health-provider response to it. The relations among these variables and their eventual combined effects on family structure and process will be better understood with continued research.

A weakness of many past studies on the differences illness makes on the family has been that family and illness were viewed as if they constitute an isolated dyad, unaffected by the responses of health care providers and the requirements of treatment. When considered, treatment was often seen as an aspect of the illness and not separated from it for purposes of practical analysis. Yet we know that variability of health provider response toward the "same" problem is the rule rather than the exception and that such variability creates widely different experiences for patients and their families. It seems, therefore, that along with the type of illness and "response style" of the family, we need always to include the response and involvement of health providers in order to appreciate the effects on the family of any illness.

Some studies are beginning to integrate more fully the role of treatment in the total picture. Recent research on the effects of kidney transplantation and the search for kidney donors provides an illustration of the powerful reverberations as available medical procedure can set off in both nuclear and extended family systems (e.g., Kemph, Bermann, & Coppolillo (1969); Fellner & Marshall (1968, 1970); Simmons, Klein, & Thornton (1973). As the scope and scale of medical technology increases, we find ourselves being forced to examine the "fallout" just as we have in other areas of powerful technological specialization and growth. In the formal sense, the problem of pollution applies to the health care industry in the same way that it applies to agriculture.

3. Family-Health Services Provider Relations

The study of the effects of treatment on the family leads naturally to a larger set of questions about all the imaginable ways that families and health care providers relate to one another. Here we are concerned about everything from the traditional house call to the logic and economics of health insurance policies, which by underwriting only individual members one by one, fail to cover families as biosocial units.

One area of enduring interest is the "doctor-patient relationship" (e.g., Balint, 1957; Blum, 1960; Bloom, 1963). Family medicine has enlarged the focus to "doctor-family" and, perhaps more representatively, to "health care team-family" since it is becoming increasingly clear that what families need and want cannot be and need not be supplied entirely or exclusively by physicians.

Serious efforts to develop family-centered health services create both challenges and threats to conventional health care providers and to the current predominant models of organizing health services. The potential for constructive change contained in the family approach may well be timely and fortunate, for there is evidence that the "old order" of health care relations is losing its viability and is coming increasingly under question (Haug & Sussman, 1969). The exclusiveness of traditional doctor-patient encounters has carried a cloak of invisibility that leads to problems around the issue of control. Having to deal with families increases the visibility of what is going on both inside and outside of the doctor's office. Maintaining the subordinate-superordinate model of health care exchanges [in which, for example, the good patient is the one who conforms and follows without question the instructions of the professional, the superordinate in the relationship, who "knows best" (Sussman, 1972)] is much more difficult when one must relate to the family as a group instead of to a single patient. Families have an unmatched stake in the health of their members and can more easily challenge "medical advice" than an individual can. This issue of increasing informational exchanges that lead to collaboration and sharing decisions by itself creates revolutionary possibilities for patterns of family-health care provider relatedness.

One widely identifiable response signaling an increased recognition of families as consumers of health services is the increase in primary health care teams whose aim is to deal with family as well as individual health care needs. Such teams, variously composed of physicians, family nurse practitioners, social workers, family health workers, behavioral scientists, nutritionists, and others, depending upon the setting and the types of problems encountered, often give the appearance of tentatively formed families themselves, and demonstrate some of the processes and traits that we identify with family and other primary group life. However, more important than the structure and composition of family health care teams is the type are quality of relationship that develops between members of the health care provider group and members of the family group. One family physician, Lynn Carmichael (1976), even suggests that the important meaning of "family" in family medicine is contained in the *relationship* between providers and patients, a relationship whose form can be like that of family relatedness, demonstrating qualities of affinity, intimacy, reciprocity, and continuity. Persons who construct a relationship characterized by these qualities may feel they are a family whether or not they share a common household or marital ties. Thus, physician and patient, health care team and family are communicants in a process of exchange that is family-like, a relationship whose success depends upon the proper exercise of reciprocal rights and obligations among the participants as well as upon utilitarian (medical) decision making.

What we may be witnessing in such a conscious redefinition of the health care process is an adaptive response to new, or at least renewed, expectations about it. It could be that if we are seriously going to get involved with peoples' lives in the health care process, we must "meet fire with fire" so to speak, engaging one group (families) with another group (health care teams) around shared problems. Cogswell's (1968a, 1968b) work certainly indicates that consumers of health care services want relationships with representatives of those services based upon a principle of exchange and reciprocity. Persons on the receiving end want more two-sided, personal, and human relationships with providers. Family medicine represents the possibility of a more balanced and humanistic model of patient-professional, family health care system relationships, whose nature provides an expansive and virtually unexplored domain for research.

Efforts to reorganize mainstream health care to engage families are most prevalent in "model family practice centers" that provide the unifying focus for residency training in family practice programs in the United States and Canada. While just beginning, programs that are undergoing the growing pains of becoming family-focused are providing a variety of experiments in staffing, problem conceptualization, and the delivery of services, which, in turn, are producing some interesting discoveries.

In one everyday function, family charts and family problem lists are enabling the reorganization of record keeping and providing a formal means of focusing attention at the family level. At the University of California at Davis, Smilkstein (1975) developed the Family Problem-Oriented Record as a means of organizing interventions around problems which are conceptually distinct from individual family member problems. Similarly, for purposes of medical charting, Medalie (1978) presents a method of constructing a family tree, documenting the essentials of a family history, and undertaking family assessment and diagnosis, which also represents the logical and pragmatic distinction between the family and the individual. The first published example of a Family-Oriented Medical Record from a community-based group practice in the United States comes from Grace, Neal, Wellock, and Pyle (1977) who keep individual records inside a surrounding family record that contains a family database and family problem list together with the individual members' problem lists.

At McMaster University Clinic in Hamilton, Ontario, conjoint family meetings are routinely offered by the family practice residents when an emotional problem is identified with one of the members. The purpose of such meetings is to look at the roles various members take in the family, to assess their methods of communication and control, to explore the family's problem-solving techniques and the resources available to them, and so on. The goal is to develop methods and tap resources within the family for dealing with problems which have traditionally been brought to the physician as an emotional complaint, or as a masked somatic or psychosomatic complaint. During the course of these family sessions, the family decides on a method of dealing with the problem and usually reports back in a few weeks. Comley (1973) was interested in whether this family approach had any effect on the pattern of overall demands for health care made by the family. He compared a sample of 42 families engaged in family sessions with an equal number of families matched for problems and utilization during the previous year, but whose members received traditional approaches of medication or individual psychotherapy. Comley found that in the year following the first conjoint session, families in the study group showed a 49% decrease in their demand for medical services while families in the contrast group showed a 10% increase. This was true even though 29 of the 42 families in the study group met only once or twice to work on the problem. Comley pursued this outcome further to be sure families in the study group were not going elsewhere for services they had previously received at the clinic. As it turned out they were not, nor were they aware of their substantial reduction in visits to the Clinic. The results further showed that for both groups the pattern of the type of complaints brought to the Clinic did not differ significantly in the year follow-up period.

A common lament among primary health care providers is that the family approach seems intriguing and makes intuitive sense, but time constraints and the lack of sufficient training forbid its systematic use. The importance of the McMaster study is that it is the first published evidence that family-centered intervention is a timesaver in the long run, and that for many common complaints, getting the family together in the health center to mobilize resources and focus on a problem is more important than worrying about the level of training of the primary care provider.

The misconception that working with families is a luxury and that organizing health care services around family units is both extravagent and unnecessary, is common. Yet the closer we look in virtually every area of health care delivery, the more it appears that ignoring the family is costly in both dollars and in the terms of treatment outcome. The issue is not simply a matter of choosing to develop an appreciation of fuller understanding of the patient's interpersonal environment. It appears that we must engage the social environment itself if health care goals are to be realized rather than subverted or left wanting. There is an axiom in Gregory Bateson's approach to human communication which states that when one is in relation to another, there is no way not to communicate (e.g., see Ruesch & Bateson, 1959, Weakland; 1965; Watzlawick, Beavin, & Jackson, 1967). We can extend this axiom to the medical domain by stating that when one gets involved with a person's health, there is no way not to get involved with his or her family, real and imaginary, past, present, and future. So the question becomes not *whether*, but *how* one chooses to get involved.

The consequences of not dealing with the family when attempting to treat a family member are becoming better known in psychotherapeutic treatment. Such consequences from other areas of concern are drawing increasing attention, e.g., from surgery (Baudry & Wiener, 1968); rehabilitation (Peck, 1974); dentistry (Kriesberg & Treiman, 1962; Bell, 1975); health maintenance (Litman, 1974b); medication (Pratt, 1973); and cooperation with medical advice (Oakes et al., 1970). On the other side, successful methods of engaging and working together with family members around a common goal appear from time to time, but need more systematic exploration and documentation. Over 20 years ago, John Clausen (Clausen et al., 1954) discovered that mothers who were given more information were more willing to participate in a polio vaccination program for their children than mothers who were given less information. When we look at Hoebel's (1975; 1976) success at modifying risk behaviors in male patients with coronary artery disease by working only with and through their wives, we catch a glimpse at how far we have come in our ability to think about the family in operational terms and to influence the health care of one family member by relating meaningfully with another member.

Another set of issues providing extensive research opportunities and important implications for changing patterns of health care can be found in family-hospital interrelations (see Ransom & Dervin, 1978). It should be pointed out, however, that excepting the needs of children in the hospital, little systematic work has been done on the problems generated when a family member must be hospitalized.

Interest in this subject has traditionally been focused on the transfer or curtailment of various personal or parental functions upon hospitalization. Parsons and Fox (1952) wrote about the "desocialization" process that occurs when a patient enters a hospital. Ordinary rights and obligations are given up as the person is confirmed in the "sick role" by medical personnel and a larger hospital system whose authority must be acknowledged, and whose rules and customs must be adhered to. On the discharge end, the problem of "resocialization" when the person leaves the hospital has also been identified and studied. Coser (1956) described a trained incapacity to readjust to home life in persons who become fully adapted to hospital routines as patients.

From the wealth of activities that take place between a family and a hospital, Bell and Zucker (1968) have abstracted a set of basic interchanges. These six dimensions of interchange are useful in organizing family-hospital observations, providing a basis to analyze the quality of the relationship, and describing it in terms of what is going on, what is missing, and where points of conflict may be expected.

Bell and Zucker start with the assertion that families and hospitals are two fundamental but quite different types of social systems engaging in periodic relation with one another within the larger community. Their points of contact, accessibility to one another, images and expectations of one another, and demands upon one another are all dimensions that can be studied. At some point, the family and the hospital share a common interest in a patient/family member. A workable relationship between the two is essential for a complete set of exchanges and for hospital-medical procedures to run smoothly. John Bell (1969) carried a similar conceptual framework to Africa and Asia where he visited more than 100 medical facilities to see what lessons other societies could provide on family-hospital relations. The result was a monograph, *The Family in the Hospital* (1969), the most extensive treatment of the subject to date.

From the vantage point of a cross-cultural perspective, Bell (1969; 1975) describes a state of disarticulation between the family and the hospital in the United States. Operationally, a state of disarticulation between the two systems is defined as a type of communication resulting in a relationship that produces undesired changes in one instead of achieving a functional relationship in which both systems maintain their own integrity. Failure to recognize basic differences in family and hospital system functioning combined with the pressures of institutional efficiency and the predominant individual orientation of modern medicine have led to the serious disarticulation emphasized by Bell. The best known symptom of this state is the "institutionalization" of the patient, a secondary or latent consequence of the treatment process shaped by the hospital. In its extreme form, the failure of family and hospital to achieve reciprocity results in the dissolution or destruction of the entire family group. As the recognition of medical-institutional iatrogenesis increases, the documentation of horrifying case illustrations no doubt will also increase.

4. The Family as Its Own Health Promoting Agency

In Part 1 of this research section it was proposed that one major dimension of family medicine is the concern with ways the family is involved in the origins and maintenance of ill health. But, "the same flame that melts the butter hardens the egg." Turning the first question around, we are interested in all the ways family membership and primary group relatedness restore, protect, and enhance health and well-being. Compared to questions raised in the other three categories outlined here, few investigations have studied the family's positive role in health. It seems today that this is a central question for the future of family medicine, and perhaps, for future forms the family itself will take.

In an extensive 5-year investigation of ischemic heart disease among 10,000 Israeli men aged 49 years and over, Medalie and Goldbourt (1976) found that anxiety and family problems played major independent roles in the development of new angina pectoris. Yet, in the same study, they also found that perceived love and support from one's wife reduced the risk of angina pectoris, *even in the presence of high risk factors, including anxiety*. This is perhaps the largest-scale documentation of a pattern of independent positive and negative family effects on a specific clinical problem.

The beneficial effects of primary group membership have long been known by sociological investigators. Durkheim (1897), followed by Miner (1922) and Sainsbury (1956), demonstrated that suicide occurs less frequently among persons embedded in families than among those who lived without such an association. In this work, membership was juxtaposed with isolation or reduced meaningful contacts. The question still remains whether, in a group of 10,000 adult Israeli males, for instance, disjunctive family relations [in the Sullivanian (1953) sense] are better than no immediate relations at all.

In thinking of family roles in good health, we can imagine a spectrum of relevant variables from socially selected exposure to risk factors at one end, to ineffable feelings of belongingness, or occupying a proper place in the world, at the other. No doubt objections will be raised to proposing explanatory variables that cannot be observed or described in operational terms. Yet it seems that simply knowing or believing or feeling something can have enormous benefits, even when that something cannot be identified or confirmed by an observer. The effects created by *meaning* must be given an important place in family medicine, a suggestion which poses no unusual problem for clinical semiotics, ethology, or general systems theory, but which creates havoc for a number of other viewpoints.

The protection from disease that accompanies differential exposure to health risks is determined by such factors as a family's place of residence, values, health, and dietary norms, and follows also from the latent consequences of social interaction patterns structured by membership in the group. Moss (1973) discusses these safeguards in order to differentiate them from other types of social processes that he proposes constitute "social immunity." Examples of social selection would include the protection from cervical cancer lent by the increased likelihood of virginity that accompanies membership in the universal family of Catholic nuns (Gagnon, 1950; Towne, 1955);

and the decreased probability of fatal automobile accidents among persons belonging to networks that discourage consumption of alcohol and driving soon after (McCarroll & Haddon, 1962). Drawing on less obvious examples, being poor may protect one from myeloid leukemia: exposure to x-rays increases the risk, so that those who can afford more medical care may be more vulnerable to this disease (Graham, 1970). Belonging to a family of lower socioeconomic status may reduce the risk of breast cancer where numerous pregnancies, nursing of children, and early menopause resulting from hysterectomy or ovariectomy are more common (Graham, 1968; Bart, 1968).

Exposure to risks through such social selection derives from one's position in networks within the larger social structure. More commonly, however, when we think about the family as a resource or as its own health promoting agency, we have in mind the variety of beneficial instrumental behaviors families engage in, particularly in response to health needs. An example of research interest in such patterns is the work of Sussman and his colleagues (e.g., Sussman, 1959; 1971; 1972; Sussman & Burchinal, 1962) on the specific roles family and kin networks play in the care and rehabilitation of disabled members. Their findings stimulated the rediscovery of the family as a resource that had largely been written off. Family and kin networks link members directly to services, provide doctoring and nursing needs, and lend financial support in time of need to a much greater degree than had been commonly assumed. Also, Pratt (1973) has shown that the family plays a a more frequent and decisive role in medication activity than we might expect if we follow the assumption that, as society becomes increasingly industrial, technical, and complex, many functions formerly performed by families become absorbed by specialized agencies. Further, she has demonstrated that family self-medication can be reasonably viewed, not as a form of deviant behavior, but as a health protective activity. As in the example of family-hospital relations discussed earlier, Pratt points out that the family and the health care system have their own separate interests, needs, and goals which build elements of conflict over decision making and control into the relationship. The family simply cannot safely delegate full responsibility for crucial health needs and decisions to outsiders. Further, to insist that representatives of the health care professions really are or can be "members of the family" is to mystify the specialized nature of the exchange (relationship) beyond all recognition.

Other examples of specific family responses to perceived health needs include discoveries by Shanas (1968), who found that the care of 75% of the elderly in an English community was wholly contained within the household; White et al. (1961) who found that about two-thirds of the 75% of the populations of the United States, England, and Wales who experience some illness or injury during a month will take care of it without professional consultation; and Alpert et al., (1967) who found in a study of a month of illnesses among low-income families that medical help was sought in only 12% of the symptoms identified by the families.

Less specific and not so obviously instrumental family functions have also been studied for their effects on health. An example is the series of studies in an Italian-American community in Roseto, Pennsylvania (e.g., Stout et al; 1964). In Roseto, the death rate from heart disease is remarkably low despite the prevalence of predisposing factors: lack of exercise, large consumption of animal fat, cigarette smoking, and high blood pressure. When compared to neighboring communities matched on risk and genetic factors, a 12-year study found the death rate from heart disease to be half that of surrounding communities, even when relatives were compared. The most striking difference—the immunizing factor—appeared to exist in the social environment. Strong family and community ties lead to many types of emotional and practical support, a sense of security and belongingness, and freedom from certain types of stresses, even while other types are present. This reminds us of the Medalie (1976) study cited earlier, in which perceived love and support offset other risk factors in the development of angina.

These long-term heart studies from Pennsylvania and Israel move beyond looking at the benefits of specific responses to health needs toward the more subtle and complex questions concerning what patterns of family and community life increase the likelihood of good health among the members. We know very little about this question, really, at least from systematic research. An ambitious effort to investigate the ways groups protect members from social stress has come from Moss (1973). Concentrating on the cognitive level, Moss develops the linkages between individual confrontations with informational incongruities, physiological responses, and disease susceptibility, and then describes how groups embody processes of resistance and immunity through blocking, reducing, or eliminating such incongruities. In other studies, we are finally coming to know something about "normal" and "healthy" families by observing directly their interaction. Kantor and Lehr (1975) and Lewis et al. (1976) have made recent significant contributions in this direction.

Service and Teaching

Looking back over the discussion of family roles in health and care, it is instructive to note that nearly all contributions by behavioral scientists mentioned here have come from theorists and basic researchers who supply ideas and information for others to use in setting policy and solving problems.

Unfortunately, very little of what is thought and discovered ever reaches policy makers or health care providers. Even when it does, such information is seldom easy to use. To make matters worse, "normal" sickness care does not assimilate easily what behavioral science has to offer. When the principal tool of a trade is a hammer, those involved ordinarily attempt to solve problems with nails. Rather than providing more nails, behavioral scientists offer other types of tools and alternative plans and problem-solving principles. Thus, a problem is that physicians cannot readily see either the relevance or the practical usefulness of what behavioral scientists produce. The result is that both groups become disappointed and mutual alienation and antagonism sets in.

Two responses aimed at reducing this persistent problem are the following. First, the role of a subgroup of behavioral scientists can be expanded to include direct patient care responsibilities. A major benefit would be to gain the perspective of both the consumer's and provider's eye view in clinical settings at the moment that care is delivered. (By the same token, physicians could, at times, take on behavioral science roles, either through research activity or by engaging in a different type of patient contact designed to expand their experience of assessment and intervention.) Second, rather than maintain the traditional line drawn between those who do research and lecture and those who provide services, a major effort could be undertaken to provide clinical faculty who combine systematic investigation and front line service.

The application of principles of family medicine provides ideal opportunities for behavioral scientists to expand their roles in these two directions. The centrality of the social environment for individual behavior, the emphasis on prevention and health education, the concern for first contact availability and care for all age groups over long spans of time, the importance of patient advocacy and linkages with specialized services and subspecialty care, and the types of problems encountered—especially chronic diseases and "diseases of living"—all combine to reshape the meaning of basic health care and redefine the requirements of education in the health professions. A new group of behavioral scientists is emerging in response to these challenges. At last, we are beginning to see the development of a lingering idea: the *clinical behavioral scientist*.

What distinguishes the modern clinical behavioral scientist from traditional roles in consultation, policy development, and community work are three features: direct patient contact, shared responsibility for the outcome of persons who seek change or relief through contacting the health care system, and payment for services rendered (in addition to/or instead of payment only for teaching or research consultation).

Such ideas and their accompanying roles for behavioral scientists are not new. They are periodically recycled in various forms, much like the interest in the family and health mentioned earlier. The term "clinical sociology" appears to have been introduced by Louis Wirth (1931) in a sense further developed by Lennard and Bernstein (1969) in *Patterns in Human Interaction: An Introduction to Clinical Sociology*, in which sociological theory and methods of investigation are applied to clinical situations. While Lennard and Bernstein's conception applied primarily to problems falling within the fields of psychiatry and clinical psychology, it can easily be extended to more general questions of health and illness and to clinical situations of all kinds. Caudill described a role for a "clinical social scientist" in 1958 as a professional person from the fields of anthropology or sociology who would combine some clinical responsibilities with the more traditional roles of teaching residents and nurses, and doing research. Cohen and Kelner (1976) draw attention to Caudill's concept and further distinguish how a clinical sociologist might differ from a medical social worker. Gouldner (1965) is another contemporary sociologist who has referred to clinical sociology in a book on applied social sciences. No doubt other sociologists have discussed the general concept.

Psychologists have experimented with a number of roles in the health care system over the years, from psychophysical testing to the modification of risk behaviors at the family level. The idea of psychologists as health professionals in general is now being worked out in greater detail. Recent discussions can be found in the American Psychological Association Journal, *Professional Psychology*, by Scholfield (1976) and Wiggins (1976) who are beginning to articulate the idea with potential roles in health maintenance organizations (HMOs). A recent American Psychological Association report by the Task Force on Health Research (1976) emphasizes the role psychology has played in basic and applied research on behavioral factors in illness and health and encourages the support and continued development of psychologists as health researchers at all levels. While the emphasis of the report is on research roles, the task force also takes the position that:

> there is a need to give serious thought to innovate programs of graduate training that will prepare psychologists to carry their expertise effectively into the general clinic, the hospital, the rehabilitation center, the community health center, and the group medical practice (APA Task Force, 1976, p. 272).

The suggestion was also made that a "suitable home" be found within APA for a core group working within the health field. Such a home was established on August 30, 1978, when the Council of Representatives of the APA approved a petition signed by some 700 charter members to establish Division 38 as the Division of Health Psychology.

No doubt suggestions and descriptions for a "clinical anthropologist" have been made in a literature with which I am less familiar. Certainly Weakland's (1977) concept of "family-somatics" embodies the viewpoint contained in this paper and, judging from his own clinical work, provides a role for anthropologists in direct contact with persons and families with the aim of working together toward solving health problems.

The suggestion that persons undertake careers in clinical behavioral science immediately raises the questions of how and where they should be trained and by whom, where they would work, and how they would later be paid for their services. Those now involved in developing this role have largely "scratched out their own specialized training," to borrow a description from the APA Task Force Report (1976). This has certainly been true in my own case. The closest available models are those of the medical social worker and some clinical psychologists and psychiatrists. The structure of formal training in these professions provides a reasonable starting point. With generous allowances for the differences between the special concerns of each discipline, a focus on general health instead of or in addition to mental health combined with field placements and internships in health care centers instead of mental health centers could provide the basis for trial training models. Graduate programs in the psychology, sociology, and anthropology of health, leading to a *clinical* doctorate, would be the result. Variety in such programs should be encouraged, but, in any case, I agree with Ficken (1974) that the clinical training involved should be in addition to and not a substitute for the traditional broad-based preparation of behavioral scientists. What is not needed is simply another trade school variety of practitioner who corners yet another share of the health care market to be defended by yet another professional guild.

Opportunities for health manpower training support, licensure, freedom of choice legislation to provide reimbursable options to consumers, and many other issues obviously need exploration and a great deal of thought. But it is now reasonable, and at last possible, that any national health policy, including insurance coverage, that is truly comprehensive and directed toward the whole person, families, and health would provide a place for clinical behavioral scientists. Furthermore, if criteria for developing such a policy should begin to include a consideration of outcome in addition to customary practice and a serious look at cost effectiveness as well as the desire to support conventional providers, the place for the role being advocated here would be further strengthened.

Outside those who have tried it, few appreciate the difficulties of behavioral scientists attempting to teach in medical settings. The problem for those who are primarily engaged in and who identify themselves with research is not as great. It seems that however antagonizing the research results sometimes turn out to be for mainstream medical care and the health professions, behavioral science researchers are of substantial value in medical centers if only because of their comparative superiority and leadership in research design and methodology. The problems of those who primarily teach, however, are enormous, and stem from several sources: from the demands inherent in the educational context of the medical center (usually a tertiary care base striving to prepare technical specialists), and from the three most relevent groups involved–the medical faculty, students, and often from their own colleagues. Explorations of these difficulties together with a reexamination of the role of behavioral science in medical education have become popular subjects. Useful discussions can be found in the December 1973 Special Issue of *Social Science and Medicine*, Hunt, 1974; Williams et al., 1974; Sluzki, 1974; Volpe, 1974; Routh & Clarke, 1976; Cohen & Kelner, 1976; and Wexler, 1976. A most penetrating analysis from a sociologist's viewpoint is provided by Jeffries, 1974.

The presence of increasing numbers of behavioral scientists in care delivery settings such as kidney dialysis units, pediatric hospitals, primary care clinics, and family practice centers is beginning to contribute examples of how services and teaching can work hand in hand. From these experiences, especially those in family practice programs (e.g., Johnson et al., 1977), a number of observations are beginning to provide the basis for consensus on several issues. These are the subject of another paper in preparation. In closing this discussion, I shall suggest only that the clinical behavioral scientist model advocated here provides a hopeful response to increasing pressure from a major prevailing issue: what and how to teach in order to make behavioral science "clinically relevent," i.e., to help health providers achieve immediate goals and to "actually demonstrate in concrete situatons that (our) knowledge and skills can improve the quality of health care" (Cohen & Kelner, 1976, p. 27).*

This approach to teaching is admittedly labor intensive and deliberately clinically biased. It also requires that "student" and "teacher" work closely together to construct the ground rules for their relationships, two by two and

*It should be pointed out that improving health care and meeting the needs of providers are demands that may or may not be compatible with one another. The potential for role conflicts of this type for the behavioral scientist is a constant problem. The question of whose definition of the problem behavioral scientists accept is discussed later in this paper.

in small groups. To someone like myself who was raised on one-way mirrors and is accustomed to being directly observed or recorded, it seems astonishing that a medical student or resident can go through his or her entire training without once being directly observed interviewing a patient. Increasing the visibility of what actually goes on inside the medical examining room is itself a great breakthrough.

Teaching around and through patient care allows the behavioral scientist to focus actively within the two dimensions that I believe provide the areas of his or her most useful contribution to primary health care providers: the application of specific techniques or the provision of basic information to work on a specific problem; and the application of alternative frameworks (viewpoints) and strategies for working on a class of problems. Both may involve the exploration and analysis of fundamental assumptions that govern how a medically trained provider thinks about and intervenes into human problems in general. In such instances, dealing with real cases and sharing responsibility for results inevitably proves to be more meaningful than dealing with hypotheticals.

The behavioral scientist as "epistemological provocateur" is a valuable and time-honored role. He or she can suggest different lenses to view the "same" everyday situation. At the very least, providers can learn to see themselves as part of the situation they are attempting to influence. When the doctor-patient encounter is viewed as a piece of social and cultural behavior; when every medical act is seen also as a political act, in the broadest sense, in terms of the statuses to which people are assigned and the ways in which the options for future behavior are delimited; when the unanticipated or latent consequences of medical intervention are learned to be recognized and respected along with the manifest ones; when the nature of learning and learning contexts are examined; when the models of human nature sustaining attitudes about motivation and patient cooperation are made explicit; when disease is viewed as a construct rather than an entity—when these sorts of issues are examined around specific and ongoing behavior rather than in the lecture hall, the basis of medical practice itself begins to change.

Comment

In closing, I would like to comment briefly on two questions likely to be raised by readers. One has to do with the proposed involvement of behavioral scientists on a larger scale and more directly in health care than has been considered before, and the other has to do with the conception and implications of the aims of family medicine itself.

If behavioral scientists are to play an increasing role in family medicine, health care, and medical education, whose agents will they be? Since every description of every situation is the product of "punctuating" the flow of experience in one way rather than some other, all descriptions can be thought of as motivated by the interests of those who provide them. Even the most simple research question or clinical intervention is framed from someone's point of view. In matters of health it is important to consider whose point of view is being adopted and whose problem is being addressed, since it cannot be assumed that complementarity, mutual interest, and mutal benefit exist among all parties involved.*

The subject of "patient compliance" provides a good illustration of the meaning of the question. Research psychologists have invested considerable effort in studying why patients do not always comply with medical advice. The issue, however, is nearly always framed from the physician's viewpoint, not the patients', as if the desirability of the consequences of compliance were identical for all concerned and beyond question. "Why do patients leave the hospital against medical advice?" and "Why do patients fail to take their medicines as prescribed?" are asked instead of, "Why do patients stay in the hospital?" and "Why do people take drugs in the first place?" Roth (1962) sees this as the management bias in social scientific research. Gold (1977) would see it as the consequence of behavioral science being subordinated to the more powerful field of medicine. Her critique (1977) is a recent contribution in a long line of explorations and warnings by social scientists about the hazards of undertaking work on medical problems.

Foster (1975) points out that there is a range of identification by behavioral scientists with different interest groups within the health care industry. Will there be a constructive balance among the viewpoints taken up? In relation to that diverse group of potential consumers of behavioral science, "Do we owe equal time"...? Or do we simply sell our skills to the highest bidder?" as Heshka (1976) so clearly puts it. Such questions, themselves very important, still suffer from too narrow a view of the behavioral scientist, a limitation of vision that grows out of the bias of the research role and out of the failure to recognize that the medical province, in the strict sense, is inappropriate and ineffective for many health problems existing today. What is growing clearer is that the key issue for health care in the next decade is not how medical intervention can be improved and increased, but how health related personal behavior can be influenced, how change in groups and institutions can be promoted, and what roles can be enacted to catalyze this

*That statement, in itself, is a contribution of behavioral science toward demystifying and identifying sources of strain in health care relations.

type of change. With this restatement, a rationale is provided to encourage behavioral scientists to expand their role from providing ideas and information for others to apply, to acting according to their own principles directly in the change-inducing process. As new roles are created, advocacy for the widest possible range of interest groups, combined with the increasing independence of behavioral scientists as providers of health services, are two safeguards against being coopted by or selling out to any one constituency.

Finally, what is to be gained by supporting the development of family medicine? The hope is that a more effective approach to addressing health problems than is presently in vogue will be constructed. One result of such an approach that is subtle but extremely important is an effect on significant learning–deutero-learning (Bateson, 1942)–in which the participants walk away from an encounter with a changed idea of what health and illness are about, what health care is, and what is expected of those joining in the process. The idea cannot be directly taught, it is a by-product of the nature of the exchange. By opening up the once invisible doctor-patient exchange to include additional persons on both sides of the relationship, both a more comprehensive approach to assessing problems and initiating change and a redistribution of control and responsibility are achieved. The "family" focus expands the ordinary view to identify ways that health is governed by our relationships with others and includes them in the process of creating change, distributing responsibility among those concerned.

Family medicine also provides a countervailing force to the "new reductionism" (Waitzkin, 1976) that characterizes contemporary debate over health care issues. The realities of health problems and health care can be distorted in a variety of ways. In the recent past may problems were reduced to failures in technological capacity, and solutions were pinned on the hope of scientific progress. Just as we began to realize that human and social problems cannot always be blamed on technology or solved by technological means, the insight was distorted. A new reductionalism arose that reduces "social issues" to "personal troubles," to borrow Waitzkin's application of C. Wright Mill's term. Poor health is now popularly described as a product of individual life-style and self-defeating personal behavior, and poor health care, in turn, is seen as the result of nonhumanistic and morally imperfect physicians. The prevalence of this view is, in part, a sign that we have lost faith in our capacity to change social relations and that our belief in one another has eroded. Unfortunately, it only legitimates a further decrease in the search for meaningful solutions to problems of health and undermines the acceptance of social responsibility for health care. The "personal troubles" perspective, when applied to matters of health, magnifies a self-reinforcing epistemological error: the denial of reciprocity and mutual interdependence that creates all subjects of our concern. It is an antiheuristic view whose perspective can lead one to think that "if we are totally responsible for our own fate, then all others in the world are responsible for their fate, and, if that is so, why should we worry about them" (Marin, 1975, p. 47). It is a back door return of Social Darwinism.

Even the new emphasis on "holistic medicine," while carrying the banners of "the whole person" and humanism, still carries the yoke of many old abstracted-individual approaches, including the hope that persons can be significantly changed without having to change the circumstances within which they live. When personal consciousness, individual responsibility, and the human will are made into principal sources of focused intervention as alternatives to significant relationships, social structures, and person-*plus*-environment systems, we have once again failed to grasp the greater half of our existence. At times, it seems to me that many of the new individual-centered technologies, from antihypertensive drugs through biofeedback and "consciousness raising" exercises, are symptoms of a widespread transpersonal defense* against having to confront the master problem, human relatedness.

Family medicine embodies an alternative approach to the problems of health and well-being that we all face. At a time when the loss of confidence in human relationships is great, family medicine turns to work with realities that conventional medical care appears to avoid or deny–personal dependence, friendship and loyalties, social cooperation, and the double-edged sword of group participation and membership–not on the grounds of moral necessity or by appeals to faith, but by establishing conceptual frameworks and strategic tools stemming from a systematic body of contextual thought and investigation.

Conclusions and Recommendations

–Family medicine is a field of inquiry and an applied discipline whose development cuts across many medical and behavioral science specialities.

–Family medicine is concerned with the health of persons in the context of their families and with families as nonreducible biosocial systems.

–The meaning of "family" in family medicine is not an entity or an institution but a type of relationship generated by primary groups or groups of intimates with a history and a future.

---

*Transpersonal defense is used here in the sense described by Laing (1971).

–Family medicine provides an alternative approach to facing problems of health and personal suffering different from that supplied by the abstracted-individual focus.

–All health care specialties can benefit from being family-centered, and family practice is likely to be the most important applied arm of family medicine.

–A broad range of behavioral scientists have been concerned with human relatedness and health and have helped to shape the field of family medicine.

–Behavioral scientists should now become fully involved in family medicine at all levels, including teaching, research, and clinical activities.

–The family should be taught in medical schools as a biosocial system alongside other systems taught at this level.

–The role of behavioral scientists involved in medical education is best served by concentrating on epistemological issues and practical problem solving in contexts of direct patient care.

–The clinical behavioral scientist role should be developed systematically; doctorates should be granted in this option in programs around the country that can support such training.

–A program of postdoctoral fellowships should be instituted that would place behavioral scientists in outstanding family practice and primary care centers as preparation for careers in family medicine.

–The public should be given free choice and direct access to those behavioral scientists who will qualify as health care providers under a national health insurance program.

REFERENCES

Alpert, J. J., Kosa, J., & Haggerty, R. T. A month of illness and health care among low-income families. *Public Health Reports*, 1967, *82*(8), 705-713.

Alpert, J. J., & Charney, E. The education of physicans for primary care. U.S. Department of Health, Education and Welfare DHEW Pub. No. (HRA) 74-3113. 1973.

American Psychological Association. Contributions of psychology to health research: Patterns, problems, and potentials. *American Psychologist*, 1976, 31(4), 263-274.

Anderson, D. A. Cystic fibrosis and family stress. *Children*, 1960, 7, 9-12.

Badgley, R. F., & Bloom, S. W. Behavioral sciences and medical education: The case of sociology. *Social Science and Medicine*, 1973, *7*, 927-941.

Balint, M. *The doctor, his patient and the illness*. New York: International Universities Press, 1957.

Bart, P. Social structure and vocabularies of discomfort: What happened to female hysteria. *Journal of Health and Social Behavior*, 1968, *9*, 188-194.

Bateson, G. Social planning and the concept of deutero-learning. In L. Bryson, and L. Finkelstein, (Eds.), *Science, Philsosophy and religion; Second symposium*. New York, Conference on Science, Philsosphy and Religion in their Relation to the Democratic Way of Life, Inc., 1942, 81-97.

Bateson, G., Jackson, D. D., Haley, J., & Weakland, J. H. Towards a theory of schizophrenia. *Behavioral Science*, 1956, *1*, 251-264.

Bateson, G. *Steps to an ecology of mind*. New York: Ballantine Books, 1972.

Bateson, G. Conference on the "ecology of mind." Family Study Station, Langely Porter Neuropsychiatric Institute. San Francisco: 1973.

Baudry, F., & Wiener, A. The family of the surgical patient. *Surgery*, 1968, *63* (3), 416-422.

Bauman, M. H., & Grace, N. Family process and family practice. *Journal of Family Practice*, 1974, *1*, 24-26.

Bell, J. E. *The family in the hospital*, Washington, D.C.: U.S. Government Printing Office, 1969.

Bell, J. E. *Family therapy*. New York: Aronson, 1975.

Bell, N. W., & Zucker, R. A. Family-hospital relationships in a state hospital setting: A structural functional analysis of the hospitalization process. *International Journal of Social Psychiatry*, 1968, *15*, 73-80.

Black, P. McL. Must physicians treat the "whole man" for proper medical care? *The Pharos*, 1976, 8-11.

Bloom, S. W. *The doctor and his patient*. New York: Russell Sage, 1963.

Blum, R. H. *The management of the doctor-patient relationship*. New York: McGraw-Hill, 1960.

Bowen, M., Dysinger, R. H., Brodey, W. M., & Basamania, B. Study and treatment of five hospitalized family groups with a psychotic member. Paper presented at the American Orthopsychiatry Association meeting. Chicago: 1957.

Carmichael, L. The family in medicine, process or entity? *Journal of Family Practice*, 1976, *3*(5), 562-563.

Caudill, W. A. The psychiatric hospital as a small society. Published for the Commonwealth Fund in Cambridge: Harvard Univeristy Press, 1958.

Chodoff, P., Freidman, S., & Hamburg, D. Stress, defenses and coping behavior: Observations in parents of children with malignant disease. *American Journal of Psychiatry*, 1963, *120*(8), 744-749.

Clausen, J. A. et al. Parent attitudes toward participation on their children in polio vaccine trials. *American Journal of Public Health*, 1954, *44*, 1526-1536.

Clausen, J. A., & Yarrow, M. (Eds.). The impact of mental illness of the family. *Journal of Social Issues*, 1955, *11*, entire issue.

Clyne, M. D. *Night Calls: A study in general practice*. London: Tavistock Publications, 1961.

Cogswell, B. E. Self-socialization: Readjustment of paraplegics in the community. *Journal of Rehabilitation*, 1968, *34*, 3.

Cogswell, B. E. Socialization into the family: An essay on some structural properties of roles. In M. B. Sussman (Ed.), *Sourcebook in marriage and the family*. Boston: Houghton Mifflin, 1968, 366-377.

Cohen, P. C. The impact of the handicapped child on its family. *Social Casework*, 1962, *43*, 137-142.

Cohen, R., & Kelner, M. Teaching behavioral science in Canadian medical schools: Some current issues. *Social Science and Medicine*, 1976, *10*(1), 23-28.

Comley, A. Family therapy and the family physician. *Canadian Family Physician*, 1973.

Cook, J. J. Family limitation subsequent to the birth of a cerebral palsied child. *Cerebral Palsy Review*, 1963, *24*, 8-9.

Coser, R. L. A home away from home. *Social Problems*, 1956, *4*, 3-17.

Crain, A. J. et al. Effects of a diabetic child on marital integration and related measures of family functioning. *Journal of Health and Human Behavior*, 1966, 7, 122-127.

D'Ary, E. Congenital defects. 1. Some findings concerning the impact on the family. *Nursing Times*, 1969, *65*, 1421-1422.

Davis, F. *Passage through crisis*. Indianapolis: Bobbs Merrill, 1963.

Debuskey, M. *The chronically ill child and his family*. Springfield, IL: Charles C. Thomas, 1970.

DeLaMata, R. G., Gingras, G., & Wittkower, E. D. Impact of sudden severe disablement of the father of the family. *Canadian Medical Association Journal*, 1960, *82*, 1015-1020.

Durkheim, E. *Le suicide*. Paris: F. Alcan, 1897.

Easson, W. M. *The dying child: The management of the child or adolescent who is dying*. Springfield, IL: Charles C. Thomas, 1970.

Ellenberger, H., Sangier, J., & Wittkower, D. Typical phases in the adaptation of a family to prolonged illness of a child. *Canadian Psychiatric Association Journal*, 1964, *9*, 322-330.

Fellner, C. Kidney donors: The myth of informed consent. *American Journal of Psychiatry*, 1970, *126*, 1245-1251.

Fellner, C., & Marshall, J. Twelve kidney donors. *Journal of the American Medical Association*, 1968, *206*, 2703-2707.

Ficken, R. A.B.S. A.M.E. Newsletter, 1974, *6*.

Foster, G. M. Medical anthropology: Some contracts with medical sociology. *Social Science and Medicine*, 1975, *9*, 427-432.

Frank, Lawrence K. *Society as the patient*. New Brunswick: Rutgers University Press, 1948.

Freeman, H. E., & Simmons, O. G. *The mental patient comes home*. New York: Wiley, 1963.

Friedman, S. B., Mason, J. W., & Hamburg, D. A. Urinary 17-hydoxycorticostoid levels in parents of children with neoplastic disease. *Psychosomatic Medicine*, 1963, *25*, 364.

Friedman, S. B., & Glasgow, L. A. Psychologic factors and resistance to infectious disease. *Pediatrics Clinics of North America*, 1966, *13*, 315-335.

Gangon, F. Contribution to the study of etiology and prevention of cancer of the cervix of the uterus. *American Journal of Obstetrics and Gynecology*, 1950, *60*, 516-522.

Geyman, J. Family Practice in Evolution: Progress, Problems, and Projections. *New England Journal of Medicine*, 1978, *298*, 593-601.

Gold, M. A crisis of identity: The case of medical sociology. *Journal of Health and Social Behavior*, 1977, *18*(2): 160-168.

Gordon, N. B., & Kutner, B. Long term and fatal illness and the family. *Journal of Health and Human Behavior*, 1965, *6*, 190-196.

Gouldner, A. W. Explorations in applied social science. In A. W. Gouldner and S. M. Miller (Eds.), *Applied Sociology*. New York: Free Press, 1965.

Grace, N. T., Neal, E. M., Wellock, C. E., & Pyle, D. D. The family-oriented medical record. *Journal of Family Practice*, 1977, *4*(1), 91-102.

Graham, S. New clues to the causes of cancer. *Transaction*, 1968, 43-48.

Graham, S. Behavioral factors associated with the etiology of physical diseases. Paper presented at the American Public Health Association meetings, 1970.

Greene, W. A., Goldstein, S., & Moss, A. J. Psychosocial aspects of sudden death. *Archives of Internal Medicine*, 1972, *129*, 725-731.

Haug, M. R., & Sussman, M. B. Professional autonomy and the revolt of the client. *Social Problems*, 1969, *17*, 153-161.

Heshka, S. Review of reflections on being useful. In M. Deutsch & H. Hornstein, (Eds.), *Contemporary Psychology*, 1976, *21*(8), 571-572.

Hoebel, F. C. Coronary artery disease and family interactions: A study of risk factor modification. a Doctoral dissertation, California School of Professional Psychology, San Francisco, 1975.

Hoebel, F. C. Brief family-interactional therapy in the management of cardiac-related high risk behaviors. *Journal of Family Practice*, 1977, *3*(6), 613-620.

Holmes, R. H., & Rahe, R. H. The social readjustment rating scale. *Journal of Psycho-*

somatic Research, 1967, *11*, 213-218.
Honegman, M. S. et al. Psychological impact of heart disease in the family of the patient. *Psychosomatics*, 1968, *9*, 34-37.
Hunt, S. M. The relationship between psychology and medicine. *Social Science and Medicine*, 1974, *8*, 105-110.
Insel, P. M., & Moos, R. H. *Health and the social environment.* Lexington, MA: Lexington Books, 1974.
Jackson, D. D. The question of family homeostasis. *Psychiatric Quarterly Supplement*, 1957, *31* (Part I), 79-90
Jackson, D. D. Family homeostasis and the physician. *California Medicine*, 1965, *103*, 239-242.
Jackson, D. D. Family practice: A comprehensive medical approach. *Comprehensive Psychiatry*, 1966, *7*, 338-344.
Jackson, D. D., & Yalom, I. Family research on the problems of ulcerative colitis. *Archives of General Psychiarty*, 1966, *15*, 410-418.
Jacobson, M. M., & Eichhorn, R. L. How farm families cope with heart disease: A study of problems and resources. *Journal of Marriage and Family*, 1964, *26*, 166-173.
Jeffries, M. Social science and medical education in Britain: A sociologic analysis of their relationships. *International Journal of Health Services*, 1974, *4*(3), 349-363.
Johnson, A. H., Fisher, J. V., Guy, L. J., Keith, J. A., Keller, A. H., & Sherer, L. M. Developing behavioral science for a family practice residency. *Journal of Family Practice*, 1977, *4*(2), 319-325.
Kiritz, S., & Moos, R. H. Physiological effects of the social environment. *Psychosomatic Medicine*, 1974, *36*, 96-114.
Kreisman, D. E., & Joy, V. D. Family response to the mental illness of a relative: A review of the literature. *Schizophrenia Bulletin*, 1974, *10*, 34-57.
Kriesberg, L., and Treiman, B. R. Dentists and the practice of dentistry as viewed by the public. *American Dental Association Journal*, 1962, *64*(806), 21.
Krush, A. G., Krush, T. P., & Lynch, H. T. Psychosocial factors in a family with a disfiguring genetic fault. *Psychosomatics*, 1965, *6*, 391-396.
Kuhn, T. S. *The structure of scientific revolution*. Chicago: University of Chicago Press, 1962.
Laing, R. D. *The politics of the family and other essays*. New York: Pantheon Books, 1971.
Laing, R. D., & Esterson, A. *Sanity, madness, and the family*. New York: Basic Books, 1964.
Lazarus, R. S. Psychological stress and coping in adaptation and illness. In Z. J. Lipowski, D. R. Lipsitt, & P. C. Whybrow, (Eds.), *Psychosomatic medicine: Current trends and clinical applications*. New York: Oxford University Press, 1977.
Lennard, H. L., & Bernstein, A. *Patterns in human interaction: An introduction to clinical sociology*. San Francisco: Jossey-Bass, 1969.
Lewis, J. M., Beavers, W. R., Gossett, J. T., & Phillips, V. A. *No single thread: Psychological health in family systems*. New York: Brunner/Mazel, 1976.
Lidz, T., Fleck, S., & Cornelison, A. R. *Schizophrenia and the family*. New York: International Universities Press, 1965.
Litman, T. J. Health care and the family: A three-generational analysis. *Medical Care*, 1971, *9*, 67-81.
Litman, T. J. The family as a basic unit in health and medical care: A sociobehavioral overview. *Social Science and Medicine*, 1974, *8*(9/10), 495-520.
Litman, T. J. Health care and the family: A three-generational study. An exploratory study conducted under Grant No. CH00167-02 from the Division of Community Health Services and Medical Care Administration, Bureau of Health Services, United States Public Health Service, 1974.

Lowenfeld, B. *Our blind children: Growing and learning with them.* Springfield, IL: Charles C. Thomas, 1964.

MacCarthy, D., & Booth, E. M. Parental rejection and stunting of growth. *Journal of Psychosomatic Research*, 1970, *14*, 259-265.

Marin, P. The new narcissism. *Harper's Magazine*, 1975, 45-56.

Marinker, M. The family in medicine. *Proceedings of the Royal Society of Medicine*, 1976, *69*, 115-124.

Martin, H. L., Lawn, J. H. & Wilkinson, A. H. The family and the fatally burned child. *Lancet*, 1968, *7568*, 628-629.

Mauksch, H. O. A social science basis for conceptualizing family health. *Social Science and Medicine*, 1974, *8*(9/10), 521-528.

Maxwell, G. M. & Gane, S. The impact of congenital heart disease upon the family. *American Heart Journal*, 1962, *64*, 449-454.

McCarroll, J. R., & Haddon, W. A controlled study of fatal automobile accidents in New York City. *Journal of Chronic Disease*, 1962, *15*, 811-826.

McClary, A. R., Meyer, E., & Weitzman, D. J. Observations on role of Mechanisms of depressions in some patients with disseminated lupus erythematosus. *Psychosomatic Medicine*, 1955, *17*, 311.

McEwan, P. J. M. The social approach to family health studies. *Social Science and Medicine*, 1974, *8*(9/10), 487-494.

Meadow, K. P. Parental response to the medical ambiguities of congenital deafness. *Journal of Health and Social Behavior*, 1968, *9*, 299-310.

Medalie, J. H. *Family medicine: Principles and application*. Baltimore: Williams and Wilkens, 1978.

Medalie, J. H., & Goldbourt, U. Angina pectoris among 10,000 men. II. Psychosocial and other risk factors as evidenced by a multivariate analysis of a five year incidence study. *American Journal of Medicine*, 1976, *60*, 910-921.

Meyer, R. J., & Haggerty, R. J. Streptococcal infections in families: Factors altering individual susceptibility. *Pediatrics*, 1962, *29*(4), 539-549.

Meyerowitz, J. H., & Kaplan, H. B. Familial response to stress: The care of cystic fibrosis. *Social Science and Medicine*, 1967, *1*, 249-266.

Miller, F. J. W. et al. *Growing-up in Newcastle-upon-Tyne*. London: Oxford University Press, 1960.

Miller, J. E. Towards a general theory for the behavioral sciences. *American Psychologist*, 1955, *10*, 513-531.

Miner, J. R. Suicide and its relation to climatic and other factors. *American Journal Hyg. Monograph Series 2*, 1922.

Minuchin, S. *Families and family therapy*. Cambridge, MA: Harvard University Press, 1974.

Minuchin, S. et al. A conceptual model of psychosomatic illness in children. *Archives of General Psychiatry*, 1975, *32*, 1031-1038.

Minuchin, S., Rosman, B. L. & Baker, L. *Psychosomatic families: Anorexia nervosa in context*. Cambridge, MA: Harvard University Press, 1978.

Moss G. E. *Illness, immunity, and social interaction*. New York: Wiley, 1973.

Mutter, A. Z., & Schleifer, M. J. The Role of psychological and social factors in the onset of somatic illness in children. *Psychosomatic Medicine*, 1966, *28*, 333.

Oakes, T. W. et al. Family expectations and arthritis patient compliance to a hand resting splint regimen. *Journal of Chronic Diseases*, 1970, *22*(11), 757-764.

Otto, R. & Mackay, I. I. Psychosocial and emotional disturbance in systemic lupus erythematosus. *Medical Journal of Australia*, 1967, *2*, 448.

Parkes, C. M., Benjamin, B. & Fitzgerald, R. G. Broken heart: A statistical study of increased mortality among widowers. *British Medical Journal*, 1969, *1*, 740-743.

Parson, T., & Fox, R. Illness, therapy, and the modern urban family. *Journal of Social Issues*, 1952, *8*(4), 31-44.

Pearse, I. & Crocker, L. *The Peckham experiment: A study in the living structure of society*. London: Allen and Unwin, 1943.
Pearse, I., & Williamson, G. S. *The case for action*. London: Faber and Faber, 1931.
Peck, B. Physical medicine and family dynamics: The dialectics of rehabilitation. *Family Process*, 1974, *13*(4), 469-480.
Pratt, L. The significance of the family in medication. *Journal of Comparative Family Studies*, 1973, *4*(Special Issue), 13-35.
Pratt, L. *Family structure and effective health behavior*. Boston: Houghton Mifflin, 1976.
Ransom, D. C. & Vandervoort, H. E. The development of family medicine: Problematic trends. *Journal of the American Medical Association*, 1973, *225*(9), 1098-1102.
Ransom, D. C. & Dervin, J. The Family, the hospital, and the family physician. In R. B. Taylor (Ed.), *Family medicine: Principles and practice*. New York: Springer-Verlag, 1978, *28*.
Ransom, D. C., & Massad, R. J. Family structure and function. In R. E. Rakel & H. F. Conn (Eds.), *Family practice: Second edition*. Philadelphia: W. B. Saunders, 1978, *2*.
Richardson, H. B. *Patients have families*. New York: Commonwealth Fund, 1945.
Roghmann, K. J., Hecht, P. & Haggerty, R. J. Family coping with everyday illness: Self reports from a household survey. *The Journal of Comparative Family Studies*, 1973, *IV*(1, Special Issue), 49-62.
Roth, J. A. Management bias in social science study of medical treatment. *Human Organization*, 1962, *21*, 47-50.
Ruesch, J. & Bateson, G. *Communication: The social matrix of psychiatry*. New York: W. W. Norton, 1951.
Routh, D. K., & Clarke, M. G. Psychology in a medical school. *Professional Psychology*, 1976, *7*(1), 94-106.
Sainsbury, P. *Suicide in London: An ecological study*. New York: Basic Books, Inc., 1956.
Schmale, A. H. The relation of separation and depression to disease. *Psychosomatic Medicine*, 1958, *20*, 259.
Schofield, W. The psychologist as a health professional. *Professional Psychology*, 1976, *7*(1), 5-8.
Schottstaedt, W. W. et al. Host factors affecting growth of B-hemolytic streptococci in the human pharynx: A pilot study. *American Journal of Medical Science*, 1958, *235*, 23.
Shanas, E. et al. *Old people in three industrial societies*. New York: Atherton, 1968.
Shands, H. C. The informational impact of cancer on the structure of the human personality. *Annals of the New York Academy of Sciences*, 1966, *125*, 883-889.
Shands, H. C. *Semiotic approaches to psychiatry*. The Hague: Mouton, 1970.
Shands, H. C., Finesinger, J. E. Cobb, S., & Abrams, R. D. Psychological Mechanisms in patients with cancer. *Cancer*, 1951, *4*, 1159-1170.
Silver, G. A. *Family medical care: A report on the family health maintenance demonstration*. Cambridge: Harvard University Press, 1963.
Silver, G. A. *Family medical care: A design for health maintenance*. Cambridge, MA: Ballinger, 1974.
Simmons, R. G. Hickey, K., Kjellstrand, C. M., & Simmons, R. L. Family tension in the search for a kidney donor. *Journal of the American Medical Association*, 1971, *215*, 909-912.
Simmons, R. G., & Klein, S. Family non-communication: The search for kidney donors. *American Journal of Psychiatry*, 1972, *129*(6), 63-68.
Simmons, R. G., Klein, S. D., & Thornton, K. The family member's decision to be a kidney transplant donor. *The Journal of Comparative Family Studies*, 1973, *IV*(1, Special Issue), 88-115.

Skipper, J. D. et al. Physical disability among married women: Problems in the husband-wife relationship. *Journal of Rehabilitation*, 1968, *34*, 16-19.

Sluzki, C. E. On training to "think interactionally." *Social Science and Medicine*, 1974, *8*(9/10), 483-485.

Smilkstein, G. The family in trouble–How to tell. *The Journal of Family Practice*, 1975, *2*(1), 19-24.

Sojit, C. M. The double bind hypothesis and the parents of schizophrenics. *Family Process*, 1971, *10*, 53-74.

Solomon, G. F. & Moos, R. H. Psychologic aspects of reponse to treatment in rheumatoid arthritis. *GP*, 1965, *32*, 113.

Solomon, G. F., & Moos, R. H. The relationship on personality to the presence of rheumatoid factor in asymptomatic relatives of patients with rheumatoid arthritis. *Psychosomatic Medicine*, 1965, *27*, 350.

Spiegel, J. P. & Bell, N. W. The family of the psychiatric patient. In S. Arieti (Ed.) *American Handbook of Psychiatry*. New York: Basic Books, Inc., 1959, *5*(1).

Spitz, R. A. *Hospitalism, psychoanalytic study of the child*. New York: International Universities Press, 1945(1).

Spitz, R. A. *Hospitalism, psychoanalytic study of the child*. New York: International Universities Press, 1947(2).

Stout, C., Morroe, J., Brandt, E. N., & Wolf, S. Unusually low incidence of death from myocardial infarction. *Journal of the American Medical Association*, 1964, *188*, 845-849.

Sullivan, H. S. *The interpersonal theory of psychiatry*. New York: W. W. Norton, 1953.

Sussman, M. B. The help pattern in the middleclass family. *American Sociological Review*, 1953, *18*, 22-28.

Sussman, M. B. The isolated nuclear family: Fact or fiction. *Social Problems*, 1959, *6*, 333-340.

Sussman, M. B. The family. In *Encyclopedia of social work*. New York: National Association of Social Workers, 1971, 329-340.

Sussman, M. B. A policy perspective in the United States rehabilitation system. *Journal of Health and Social Behavior*, 1972, *13*(2), 152-162.

Sussman, M. B., & Burchinal L. Kin family network: Unheralded structure in current conceptualizations of family functioning. *Marriage and Family Living*, 1962, *24*, 231.

Sussman, M. B. & Slater, S. B. Reappraisal of urban kin networks: Empirical evidence. Paper presented at the Annual Meeting of the American Sociological Association. Los Angeles: 1963.

Towne, J. E. Carcinoma of the cervix in nulliparous and cellibate women. *American Journal of Obstetrics and Gynecology*, 1955, *69*, 600-613.

Turk, J. Impact of cystic fibrosis on family functioning. *Pediatrics*, 1964, *34*(1), 67-71.

Vandervoort, H. E., & Ransom, D. C. Undergraduate education in family medicine. *Journal of Medical Education*, 1973, *48*, 158-165.

Van Heijingen, K. Psychodynamic factors in acute myocardial infarction. *International Journal of Psychoanalysis*, 1966, *47*, 370-374.

Vaughn, D. H. Families experiencing a sudden unexpected infant death. *Journal of the Royal College of General Practice*, 1968, *16*, 359-367.

Volpe, R. Behavioral science theory in medical education. *Social Science and Medicine*, 1975, *9*(8/9), 493-500.

Waitzkin, H. Review of medical nemesis: The expropriation of health by Ivan Illich. *Contemporary Sociology*, 1976, *5*(4), 401-404.

Watzlawick, D., Beavin, J., & Jackson, D. *Pragmatics of human communication*. New York: W. W. Norton, 1967.

Weakland, J. Communication and behavior: An introduction. *American Behavioral Scientist*, 1965, *10*(8), 1-3.

Weakland, J. H. Family somatics–A neglected edge. In Watzlawick and J. H. Weakland (Eds.), *The interactional view*. New York: W. W. Norton, 1977.

Wexler, M. The behavioral sciences in medical education: A view from psychology. *American Psychologist*, 1976, *31*(4), 275-283.

White, K. K., Williams, T. F., & Greenberg, B. G. The ecology of medical care. *The New England Journal of Medicine*, 1961, *265*(18), 885-891.

Wiggins, J. G. The psychologist as a health professional in the health maintenance organization. *Professional Psychology*, 1976, *7*(1), 9-13.

Wilden, A. *System and structure: Essays in communcation and exchange*. London: Barnes & Noble (distributed in the U.S.A. by Harper & Row, Barnes & Nobel [Import] Division), 1972.

Williams, I. et al. The teaching of behavioral sciences in the family medicine residency programs in Canada and in the United States. *Social Science and Medicine*, 1974, *8*(11/12), 565-574.

Williamson, G. S., & Pearce, I. *Biologists in search of material: An interim report*. London: Faber & Faber, 1938.

Wirth, L. Clinical sociology. *American Journal of Sociology*, 1931, *37*, 49-66.

Wynne, L. C., Ryckoff, I. M., Day, J. & Hirsch, S. Pseudo-Mutuality in the family relations of schizophrenics. *Psychiatry*, 1958, *21*, 205-220.

Zabarenko, R. N. Merenstein, J. & Zabarenko, L. Teaching psychological medicine in the family office practice. *Journal of the American Medical Association*, 1971, *218*, (3), 392-396.

FAMILY MEDICINE AND HOLISTIC HEALTH: AN ANALYTIC ESSAY

Kris Jeter, PhD

Throughout this century, medicine has bureaucratized and commercialized itself under the auspices of science and in the name of helping the sick. The inevitable result has been a depersonalization and growing separation between medicine and families. Two movements have emerged and blossomed to once again blend medicine with the individual and the family–family medicine and holistic health.

General practitioners declined in number due to the reactions of the AMA to the Flexner Report, one of which was a request to state legislators for licensure laws to regulate practitioners of medicine. Abraham Flexner who had been commissioned by the Carnegie Foundation to examine medical education, described medical schools he investigated as "dirty," "miserable," "utterly wretched" "very weak," and "wholly inadequate." Flexner recommended that medical education be closely associated with universities, where training in the basic sciences and clinical experience and research could be emphasized. Many medical schools found the new laws and the economics of the depression detrimental to their existence. With the schools that remained, specialization became vogue.

In the 1950s, the AMA, aware of the public concern about fragmented medicine, and the overspecialization and maldistribution of physicians in the country, encouraged the increase in the numbers of medical school graduates entering general family practice. In the 1960s, eight 2-year pilot residencies in family medicine were established. In 1964, the Ad Hoc Committee on Education for Family Practice, chaired by William R. Willard, MD, was formed by the AMA's Council on Medicine Education. Its report, "Meeting the Challenge of Family Practice," was approved by the AMA House of Delegates 2 years later. In 1966, the Millis and the Folsom Reports provided additional support for the fledgling family medicine. In 1969, family practice was recognized as the 20th medical specialty. The American Academy of Family Physicians did not "grandparent" physicians, but rather had all candidates sit for board exams and recertification examinations every 6 years.

Dr. Jeter resides at 800 Paper Mill Road, Newark, DE 19711.

Marriage & Family Review, Vol. 4(1/2), Spring/Summer 1981

Gayle Stephens has termed family medicine as "counter-culture." Its mandate is to provide individuals and families with an assessment of a clinical event, a treatment of an uncomplicated illness, and a referral when necessary. This interface of family and medicine is delicate. Raymond Duff recently advised physicians reading the *New England Journal of Medicine* that "taking the values of patient and family into account systematically from birth to death may be the only way to achieve the first goal of medicine: Do no harm." Jack Froom and Melville Rosen urged family physicians to study and to research "the family as a unit of diagnosis and treatment." He continues, "The tasks are complex and require new tools, strategies, and innovative research design. It is research of this kind, however, that can result in the integration of the family into family practice."

Meanwhile, the holistic health movement which was external and even antagonistic to formalized medicine gained strength. Folk medicine had always existed in the United States, being brought with each successive wave of immigration and then diluted with succeeding generations. Nonphysicians explored different disciplines, folk medicine, and systems of treatment used in non-Western societies in their search for answers to health questions.

Moshe Feldenkrais, physicist and Black Belt judo master, was determined to mend himself when told by doctors that recovery from his knee injury was not likely. He studied subjects such as anatomy, biochemistry, neurophysiology, psychology, and yoga to learn to heal himself. Eventually he learned how to use his permanently injured knee correctly. His studies and experience is expressed in a theory that the way a person moves and stands involves a wide array of neural impulses which is part of the brain's normal functioning of feeling, sensing, space orientation, and thinking. A person who changes movement changes the brain's wave pattern. His first book, *Body and Mature Behavior*, was published in 1949.

Wilhelm Reich, psychoanalyst and disciple of Sigmund Freud, became respected for his work in character analysis and human sexuality. He expanded this into a theory of orgone energy, a name for a universal preatomic energy derived from the words "organism" and "orgasm." Reich developed his theory of orgone energy into physical methods to open up energy blocks and allow energy to flow through the body. The expansion of his theories into agriculture, biology, medicine, meteorology, and pathology stirred controversy among biologists, physicians, psychologists–and the federal government. He died in 1957 after severe attacks on his theory and research.

Biologist O. Hans Selye's publications during the 1950s associated biochemical mechanisms and stress with "diseases of stress" and "diseases of adaptation." He interpreted the laws that regulate the body's resistance to injury and assist the body to maintain life during stress.

Feldenkrais, Reich, Selye, and others provided writings highly criticized at their publication, yet fascinating to people re-earthing their work at a later date. One work accepted by the medical establishment and by lay people developed the idea of psychological impact on health. Arnold A. Hutschnecker, a Berlin-trained internist, wrote *The Will to Live* in 1951. Thirty years, 15 printings, and numerous translations and condensations later, Hutschnecker's book still reads clear, direct, and profound.

People have biological will to live, a mission and goal to life. Life emergencies can trigger a "fight or flight" action which may become a habit and eventually wear down a specific body organ and system and, ultimately, the person. Illness may be a needed respite from problems, an unconscious way to influence others and change their behavior, and a way to vent hostility. By recognizing her or his feelings, avoiding becoming "run down," and changing our emotional reactions to negative situations we can recreate "the will to live."

All of these philosophies comprising the holistic health movement have one thing in common—a proposition that life-style creates health. The derivation of the word "health" is from the Old English word, "health," meaning wholeness. The emphasis of holistic health movements is not on disease (lack of ease) but rather on the maintenance of wholeness of a person, family, and culture. Christopher Popenoe's *Wellness* presents an extensive annotated bibliography of books on various holistic health philosophies.

One of the therapies of the 1970s gaining wide acceptance and attempting to unite family therapy, formal medicine, and holistic health movements was developed and continued at the Cancer Counseling and Research Center by radiation oncologist O. Carl Simonton and psychotherapist Stephanie Matthews-Simonton. The underlying philosophy of their therapy is that each person participates in one's health through personal actions, attitudes, beliefs, and feelings. This therapy is suggested to be in conjuction with chemotherapy and it has developed a wide group of followers—both inside and outside of traditional medicine. The Cancer Counseling and Research Center recommends the following reading list: *Getting Well Again*, *The Will to Live*, *Cancer Self-Help Education*, and *The Nature of Personal Reality*.

In their book, *Getting Well Again*, the Simonton's present an introduction to their philosophy. There are four steps of a psychological process that frequently precedes the onset of cancer.

1. People who decide as children to react in a habitual pattern may limit coping mechanisms in later life.

2. The individual reacts to many stress events, often the death of a family member or friend, in the past 6 to 18 months.

3. The person can identify no way to cope and feels helpless and hopeless.
4. The person adapts a rigid, static, and unchanging stance.

Positive attitudes toward the treatment more significantly predict the response to treatment than does the severity of the disease. Cancer needs to be considered as a disease that is not necessarily fatal when the body's own defenses in conjunction with medical treatment work against cancer.

The Simontons suggest two models of therapy—Self Assistance and Psychological Intervention. These are charted in Table I and are discussed below.

1. *Relaxation and Imagery*. The basis of the Self Assistance model is relaxation and imagery three times a day. Mike Samuels', MD and Nancy Samuels' classic *Seeing with the Mind's Eye* indicates that the "human mind is a slide projector with an infinite number of slides stored in its library, an instant retrieval system and an endlessly cross-referenced subject catalogue. . . . Meditation clears and concentrates the mind; visualization puts an image in it which can profoundly affect the life." The Simontons suggest that relaxation, meditation, and imagery can increase energy and decrease pain. Because images exist before words, mental imagery is highly personal symbolic. Effective images generally contain confused, weak cancer cells fought by a strong powerful treatment. Chemotherapy usually touches all cells and the healthy cells repair themselves quickly. The white blood cells symbolic of one's inner recovery reserves are aggressive, capable, eager to fight, intelligent, strong, sufficient in number, quick to "search and destroy" cancer cells, and victorious. The dead cancer cells are flushed out of the body in a natural process. The image ends with a picture of the person healthy and obtaining

Table I

Simonton's Models of therapy

Self Assistance	Psychological Intervention
1) Relaxation and Imagery	1) 6-18 months Prior to Diagnosis
2) Physical Exercise	2) Early Life Decisions
3) Nutrition	3) Secondary Gains
4) Goals—Quality of Life	4) Family Issues
5) Support System	5) Current Issues
6) Play	6) Redefine Life

life goals and purposes. Imageries are easily formulated to combat other diseases and chronic disabilities. Such can also be used to maintain wellness of a non-ill or diseased person.

2. *Physical Exercise*. Physical exercise is a nonspecific antidepressant. It increases flexibility in the self-acceptance concept, self-sufficiency, and modes of thinking. People schedule time to exercise and give attention to their body. People exercising more than 35 minutes a day may feel a calm highness. Fatigued muscles have been shown to decrease tumor growth.

3. *Nutrition*. Nutrition is part of one's complex belief system constructed by culture, education, and family influences. The therapist must work with the client to separate guilt from the effect.

4. *Goals–Quality of Life*. Victor Frankl in *The Meaning of Life* discusses dramatically the evidence of life goals in concentration camp survivors. The Simontons indicate that setting goals that satisfy personal and physical needs builds positive recovery expectations, expresses confidence in one's capabilities, constructs a positive self-image, and focuses energy.

5. *Support System*. The support system is most important; in fact, people actually know more people than they first imagine. This author teaches natural networking and asks workshop participants to identify persons who fill various types of needs: support, challenge, and information, for instance. People often anticipate the reactions of their friends and acquaintances before approaching them for advice. The importance of networking is further illustrated by the fact that Burnout is more of a possibility when professional, personal, and spiritual support comes entirely from one person.

6. *Play*. We all know the saying, "All work and no play makes Jack and Jill dull," and it appears also to make Jack and Jill disease prone. Play can promote uninhibited expression of feelings and thoughts, and cooperative rather than aggressive, competitive play has been found to be positive reinforcing. The major benefit for cancer patients of play can be a loss of pain during and after a play activity entered into with full concentration.

Substantiation of the effect of play on health is ancient and currently popular. The Bible advises that "a merry heart doeth good like a medicine." Physician Raymond A. Moody, Jr. traces the history of health and humor in *Laugh after Laugh: The Healing Power of Humor*. Health professionals are urged to diagnose humor status of clients and to be aware of the positive and negative consequences of humor.

Norman Cousins, editorial chair of the *Saturday Review* and senior lecturer at the School of Medicine, University of California, contends in *Anatomy of an Illness* that physicians are to provide psychological support and laying on of hands, rather than tools. In 1964, Cousins was faced with a life-threatening disease of disintegrating connective tissue of the spine (ankylosing spondylitis) and cured himself by viewing Candid Camera and Marx Brothers films, reading E. B. and Katharine White's *Subtreasury of American Humor* and Max Eastman's *The Enjoyment of Laughter*, and taking Vitamin C.

Psychological intervention takes a minimum of 1 year and usually 2 years; to contract that length of time with a therapist gives the client hope of conquering a life-threatening disease. The disease is incorporated into daily life and although it is not necessary to resolve psychological problems for a change in the course of the disease to occur, it is important that meanings to life be assigned which will in turn rekindle the will to live.

1. *Six to Eighteen Months Prior to Diagnosis*. Clients map out the stresses which faced them 6 to 18 months prior to diagnosis of their disease. Usually, there is a death of a loved one, but there are also numerous stresses which may be negative or positive and which precipitate a feeling of helplessness and hopelessness in the client. Life becomes unmanageable and even coping is difficult.

2. *Early Life Decisions*. Early life decisions tend to be made from birth till age 6 or 12. These decisions are mental ways to deal with problems—to get to an end or to avoid consequences. Because of their abbreviated chain of thought and repetition, decisions become habitual and hard to change. The person adapts a rigid, static, and unchanging stance. Decisions need to be identified and permission granted to the client with therapist protection to change.

3. *Secondary Gains*. Secondary gains are the benefits gained from being ill. Being sick is an internal sabotage which releases a person from a life-style. Because a person cannot be sick and get well, clients are to identify their secondary gains and be well. The therapist serves as a role model. The therapist and clients are to ask themselves at the onset of a cold, flu, setback, etc., "What would I do if a long-term illness set on?" and then do it. Symptoms will often go away.

4. *Family Issues*. Family issues are frequently evident. Therefore, families should accompany the client to at least one session, and there should be several marital meetings. A common family issue is the drama triangle in which family members assume the persecutor, victim, and rescuer roles. Patients are to ask directly what they want and family members are to ask the patient what is wanted. A family vs. patient stance which is often accompanied by resentment and a secret death wish may be stopped by encouraging all family members to get their needs met.

5. *Current Issues*. Current issues concern the client's day-to-day feelings about the disease itself. Cancer is so disruptive that all the sessions could be

focused on current issues; thus, it is preferable to handle current issues after the other psychological interventions are attempted. The underlying cause for the disease may be seen in current issues.

6. *Redefine Life*. Life and death are to be considered. What would the client want to do and be if born again? It is possible to change on earth without death, though patient may feel that death is inevitable and an acceptable choice. Telling the family and therapist of this choice may facilitate a rapid, natural movement to death without pain and hospitalization. The way that the patient acts during the last major crisis may indicate the quality of death, which relates to communication.

A relative, yet alternative therapy is offered by the Center for Attitudinal Healing in Tiburon, California, whose philosophy is based on *A Course in Miracles*. Gerald G. Jampolsky, MD and Pat Taylor work with children who face life and death. Healing is defined as being happy, loving, peaceful, and living in the present. *There Is a Rainbow Behind Every Dark Cloud* is an excellent book of drawings and words written by 11 of their clients.

The late Orville E. Kelly has written *Make Today Count* and *Until Tomorrow Comes* and founded Make Today Count, an organization of over 200 chapters which counsels cancer patients, their friends, families, and health professionals. The most potent force against cancer is a day-to-day commitment to life. Practical considerations of coping are suggested.

Getting patients and families to take charge of themselves, and therefore their illness, and recognizing the individual's or family's role in triggering or exacerbating the condition is in consonance with family medicine's ideology and practice. In this era and those to come, the management of chronic illness and disease of an aging population will be a priority function of the medical care system. This increase in incidence is a function of the changing demographic profile of the U.S. population. Taking charge of oneself and one's problems and using the family physician as facilitator, mediator, and expert in breadth is requisite for the mental and physical health of the practitioner, patients, and families.

REFERENCES

Achterberg, J. Simonton, O. C., & Simonton-Matthews, S. *Stress, psychological factors, and cancer: An annotated collection of readings from the professional literature*. Fort Worth, Texas: Cancer counseling and research center, 1976.

Albright, P., & Albright, B. P. (Eds.). Body, mind and spirit: The journey toward health and wholeness. Brattleboro, VT: The Stephen Greene Press, 1980.

Cancer self-help education. Saratoga, California: Health education programs, 1977.

Boston Women's Health Collective. *Our bodies, ourselves*. New York: Simon & Schuster, 1973. (Revised, 1976).

The Center for Attitudinal Healing. *There is a rainbow behind every dark cloud*. Millbrae, CA: Celestial Arts, 1978.

Cousins, N. *Anatomy of an illness as perceived by the patient: Reflections on healing and regeneration*. New York: W. W. Norton and Co., 1979.
Duff, R. Care in childbirth and beyond. *New England Journal of Medicine*, 1980, *302* (12): 685-686.
Feldenkrais, M. *Body and mature behavior: A study of anxiety, sex, gravitation and learning*. Tel Aviv, Israel: ALEF, 1949. Now New York: International Universities Press, 1975.
Eastman, M. *The enjoyment of laughter*. Johnson reprint of 1937 edition. New York: Johnson Reprint Company, 1971.
Flexner, A. Medical education in United States and Canada. A Report to the Carnegie Foundation for the Advancement of Teaching. New York: Carnegie Foundation Bulletin No. 4, 1910.
Frankl, V. E. *Man's search for meaning: An introduction to logotherapy*. New York: Beacon Press, 1959, 1963.
Foundation for Inner Peace and Coleman Graphics. *A course in miracles*. Melville, NY, 1977.
Froom, J., & Rosen, M. G. The family in family medicine research. *Journal of Medical Education*, January 1980, *55*, 60-62.
Hill, A. (Ed.). *A visual encyclopedia of unconventional medicine*. New York: Crown Publishers, 1979.
Hutschnecker, A. A. *The will to live*. New York: Prentice-Hall, 1951.
Kelly, O. E. *Until tomorrow comes*. New York: Everest House, 1979.
Kelly, O. E. *Make today count*. New York: Dell Publishing Co., 1975.
Moody, R. A. *Laugh after laugh: The healing power of humor*. Jacksonville, FL: Headwaters Press, 1978.
National Commission on Community Health Services. *Health is a community affair: The Fokom report*. Cambridge, MA: Harvard University Press, 1966.
National Commission on Community Health Services. *The graduate education of Physicians: The Millis report*. Chicago, IL: The American Medical Association, 1966.
National Commission on Community Health Services. *Meeting the challenge of family practice: The Willard report*. Report of the ad hoc committee on education for family practice. Chicago, IL: The American Medical Association, 1966.
Popenoe, C. *Wellness*. Washington, DC: Yes, Inc., 1977.
Reich, W. *Character analysis*. London: Vision Press, 1950.
Reich, W. *Selected writings*. New York: Farrar, Straus, and Cudahy, 1960.
Roberts, J. *The nature of personal reality: A Seth book*. Englewood Cliffs, NJ: Prentice-Hall, 1974.
Samuels, M. & Samuels, N. *Seeing with the mind's eye*. New York: Random House, Inc., 1975.
Selye, H. *Stress without distress*. New York: Lippencott, 1974.
Simonton, O. C. & Simonton-Matthews, S. *Getting well again*. Los Angeles. J. P. Tarcher, Inc., 1978.
Stephens, G. G. The intellectual basis of family practice. *The Journal of Family Practice*, *2*(6): 423-28, 1975.
Stephens, G. G. Reform in U.S.: Its impact on medicine and education for family practice. *Journal of Family Practice*, *3*: 507-512, 1976.
White, E. B. & White, K. S. *Subtreasury of American humor*. New York: Capricorn Books, 1962.
Willard, W. R. (see National Commission on Community Health Services)
Willard, W. W. Family centered health care. Paper delivered at Pennsylvania State University, State College, PA, April 8, 1980.

GOING THROUGH MEDICAL SCHOOL AND CONSIDERING THE CHOICE OF FAMILY MEDICINE: PRESCRIPTION OR ANTIDOTE?

Hans O. Mauksch, PhD
Edward Brent, PhD
J. Timothy Diamond, PhD
Susan Elder

Among recognized medical specialties, family medicine is a rather recent addition to the map of medical careers. Taking American Medical Association approval as an index of institutionalization, family medicine is just about 10 years old. Its history and its current place within the profession of medicine link the emergence of this specialty to a collective assertion of concern with primary and continuing care but also to an attempt by certain status-deprived segments of medicine—largely from the struggling "general practice" sector—to claim new meaning, new vehicles, and new devices for upward mobility within the profession (Mauksch, 1974; Lewy, 1977). To some, family medicine represents a deliberate move towards a professionally and scientifically-based approach to the integration of health and illness, with a holistic view of the patient as an individual and as member of a family. This is, in fact, a radical challenge to the individualistic, biopathological disease-orientation of traditional medicine. To others, the emergence of Family Medicine has been primarily a reaffirmation of simple and basic humane interests in opposition

---

Dr. Mauksch is Professor of Sociology and Professor of Family and Community Medicine, University of Missouri, Columbia, MO 65212. Dr. Brent is Assistant Proffesor of Sociology and of Family and Community Medicine, University of Missouri at Columbia. Dr. Diamond is affiliated with The Program on Women, 617 Noyes, Northwestern University, Evanston, IL 60201. Ms. Elder is Associate Director for Plan Development of the Area II Systems Agency, PO Box 128, Moberly, MO 65270.

The authors wish to acknowledge the double contribution of Jack Colwill who, as principal investigator of the Project HEW 07-D-00000-05-D, "Physicians for Rural Missouri," made this research possible and whose instrument provided the methodology on which this paper is based. M. Susan McAllister would have been one of the authors of this paper had she remained at this institution. Her coordination of data gathering and analysis and her contribution to the development of the project are greatly appreciated. The authors, however, take sole responsibility for the content of this paper.

to trends in a profession which has incurred lessened emphasis on human contact as price for gaining control over disease through technology and laboratory resources.

This new speciality clearly has its controversial components. The rhetoric of family medicine and its coverage by the mass media have served as a readily available symbol for a new version of personalized medicine. For some, this specialty is a move into a new direction of sophisticated caring, while to others it symbolizes a return to old-fashioned virtues of human concern. Within the health field itself, family medicine has evoked controversy. Its very existence has visibly influenced certain specialties such as internal medicine and pediatrics; one consequence is the trend of developing programs in primary care within these disciplines. In some states, legislatures have voted funds specifically earmarked to support family medicine, frequently governed by the perception that fostering family medicine is tantamount to providing physicians for rural America and other heretofore medically underserved areas.

The spectrum of images identified with family medicine ranges from appearing as the great hope of holistic concerns in health care to being labeled a short-lived fluff and fashion. Questions need to be raised about how this new specialty fares when medical students choose their careers. Anticipatory perceptions and interests, held at the point of entry into medical school, need to be explored. These views and preferences must be monitored as they are exposed to the various socializing influences of the medical school career.

A longitudinal study of medical student career choices, conducted at a midwestern state university, suggests certain suggestive insights into this issue. Although this study is designed to explore the entire range of specialty choices by medical students and to examine the factors underlying the selection of rural or urban practice sites, certain initial findings are specifically applicable to the choice of family medicine. Briefly, the design of the study involves the administration of a number of data collection instruments to medical students at the beginning of their first and second years, and then again at the end of their fourth year (Liccione & McAllister, 1974). Among the instruments used is the Colwill Medical Specialty Perception Inventory, which was administered at the end of the first year and at the end of the fourth year of the students' progression through the medical school. During the third and fourth years of this progression, in-depth interviews were conducted with each student. It is during this time that students rotate through eight-week clinical blocks of each major medical subspecialty. The interviews were systematically distributed to be associated with the range of clinical blocks. Each student was interviewed in connection with one of the blocks in his or her rotation; one interview before and one after the designated block. The first of these interviews seek to tap expectations about the forthcoming clinical experience, thus providing information about the student's stance toward whatever encounters and influences may be ahead. The interview conducted after the clinical block seeks to ascertain the implications of the recent experience for the student's choice of specialty, location, and style of practice. This methodology is derived from the assumption that the consequences of environment become significant through their interaction with the student's anticipation, definitions, and ongoing processes of choice and self-management.

The data reported in this paper are based on an analysis of the findings from the first of the three classes studied. The suggestive nature of initial findings and their implications for the need to understand the medical school environment gave rise to this paper. From the point of view of the data themselves, they have to be understood as representing early, heuristic results subject to further refinement and development, particularly after the analysis of the two subsequent classes has been completed.

Before reporting the findings selected for this paper a few words are in order about the medical school in which these data were collected. The administration of this medical school has made a public commitment to stress the education of physicians devoted to primary care, to family medicine, and to practice in rural areas. Admission practices, educational philosophy, and a formal statement by the medical faculty are explicitly committed to rural and to primary care and to support the school's program in family medicine.

Choosing Family Medicine

For purposes of this paper three questions are asked: Are there characteristics which differentiate students who choose family medicine from those who indicate an interest in other medical careers? Do such choices expressed at the outset of the medical school experience have significance for later decisions? What happens to first year career preferences as students progress through medical school?

Table 1 shows the anticipated career choices of 45 first year medical students and their choices 4 years later at the end of their medical school career. This table includes students who (either in the first year or at the end of the fourth year) had chosen family medicine or specialties other than family medicine or internal medicine.[1] According to Table 1, 26 of these 45

[1] Students who had indicated a choice of internal medicine either during the first year or in the fourth year are omitted from this table, since early analyses suggested that there might be ambiguity about the meaning of internal medicine, thus diminishing the sharp distinctions which are being tested.

TABLE 1

SPECIALTY CHOICES OF MEDICAL STUDENTS
AT YEAR 1 AND YEAR 4

Choice at Year 4	Choice at Year 1		Total at Year 4
	Family Medicine	Other Specialities	
Family Medicine	16	4*	20
Other Specialities	13	12	25

*Because there are so few cases in this cell, it is not included in subsequent analyses.

students reported preference for family medicine at the beginning of their first year in medical school. Of these 26, one-half (13) continued this commitment and chose to pursue a career in family medicine at the end of the fourth year. Of the 16 students who had indicated career choices in other specialties at the beginning of their first year, 12 actually did so, while only four, after 4 years, changed their mind towards a career in family medicine. The subsequent tables contain no statistical analyses with regard to these four students since their number is too small for statistical treatment. The direction of data, however, will be indicated in the text when appropriate.

Table 1 raises several questions. It is clear from these data that recruitment into family medicine seems to be linked to a proclivity in this direction based on pre-medical school interests and orientations. If this pattern is borne out by further research, recruitment into family medicine calls for a focus on pre-medical populations. Table 1 further suggests questions about possible differences between those who move from an early interest in family medicine to other medical career choices and those who persist in a family medicine career. Are these two populations different? Possibly most significant are questions to be raised about the factors which seem to move medical student orientation from family medicine to other specialties.

In order to examine selected characteristics of these students this paper utilizes data based on the Colwill Medical Specialty Perception Instrument (Cullison, Reid, & Colwill, 1976). This instrument involves a battery of 21 statements which the respondent is asked to judge on a five-point scale with regard to himself or herself and also as applied to a number of medical specialties. The scale applied to oneself is always administered at a time different from the day when data are gathered on the perceptions of medical specialties. The sensitivity of this instrument has been described by Edward Brent (1977).

A factor analysis of these perceptions was performed to determine the underlying constructs measured by these variables (Harman, 1960). The factor analysis of the Colwill Medical Specialty Perception Instrument produced five factors accounting for 61.8% of the variance. These factors in order of decreasing variance explained are (1) care, including characteristics such as compassion, humility, and personal warmth; (2) science, including characteristics such as intelligence, ability to conceptualize, and desire for intellectual challenge; (3) cure, including characteristics such as satisfaction from working with acute emergencies; (4) status, including both desire for income above the average MD and desire for prestige in the community; and (5) outside interests, including the single item interests outside of medicine (Brent, 1977, p. 5).

In examining whether the data shed any light on the changes in specialty choices from year one to year four as reported in Table 1, the data on self-perception were examined as were the data showing the perception of family medicine by these four groups. As other studies (Mauksch, 1960) have reported, data on self-perception tend to be more stable than data describing perception of professional roles. Thus, examination of the data on self for the four groups identified in Table 1 revealed no noticeable changes for four of the five factors during the medical school years. On the other hand, the factor "care" produced suggestive findings.

The mean scores for "care" indicate that already at year two there are differences between those who end up in family medicine and those who will three years later choose other specialties. Table 2 and Figure 1 show this finding which presages final choices rather than, as one might expect, reflecting the preferences held at the time data were gathered. The difference between the scores of those who stayed in family medicine and those who shifted from initially preferring family medicine to another medical specialty was not significant at year two [$t(24) = 1.56$] but was significant by year four [$t(27) = 3.57, p < .005$, 1-tailed]. Figure 1 shows graphically the findings supported in Table 2. It is clear that notwithstanding the small numbers, a potentially significant pattern is suggested. The final choice at the end of the medical school career seems to determine the grouping of the four pairs of scores on the factor care. The potential importance of this factor as having

TABLE 2

SELF-PERCEPTIONS ON THE FACTOR OF CARE AT YEARS 2 AND 4 BY CHOICE OF MEDICAL SPECIALTY

		Year 2	Year 4
$FM\text{-}FM_2$ [a]	$\bar{X}$	36.05	37.86
	N	13	16
	S	3.99	3.83
$FM\text{-}O_2$	$\bar{X}$	33.30	32.86
	N	13	13
	S	4.61	3.35
$O\text{-}FM_2$	$\bar{X}$	37.06	37.14
	N	4	4
	S	3.14	5.59
$O\text{-}O_2$	$\bar{X}$	34.10	32.15
	N	11	12
	S	6.58	5.99

[a]Notation defined in text.

predictive significance is suggested not only by the differences between the scores but also by their direction. Choosing other specialties seems to lower those perceptions of oneself which comprise the factor care, particularly for those who had already initially eschewed family medicine. By contrast, the score on care increases for those who end up choosing family medicine, particularly among those for whom this was a choice throughout medical school. For the purpose of this paper these findings only raise questions. Answers will have to await the analysis of a larger body of data and the testing of these findings in other settings and with other medical student populations.

In Table 3 and Figure 2 attention turns to the mean perception score of family medicine. Table 3A reports the perception of those students who chose family medicine at their second as well as at their fourth year. Table 3B contains comparable data for students whose choice was other specialties throughout their medical school experience. For those students who maintained their choice of family medicine, the findings indicate that there are no significant changes in their perception of family medicine. On the other hand, there are significant changes in three of the five factors in the perception of family medicine by students choosing other specialties. The latter students, in their fourth year, perceived family medicine to be lower on care, cure, and outside interests. Although not significant, the score for science also dropped. Likewise, for those students who switched from family medicine to other specialties, the scores for care, science, cure, and outside interest dropped, although not enough to yield statistical significance.

In the study quoted above, Edward Brent (1977) demonstrated that each of these factors is positively valued by medical students. Hence, these declining scores indicate that during their exposure to the medical school socialization, students ultimately choosing other specialties developed progressively less favorable perceptions of family medicine. These findings add to the argument for the need of a better understanding of the medical school as a factor influencing career choices.

Figure 1

PERCEPTION OF SELF (FACTOR CARE ONLY)
AT YEAR 2 AND YEAR 4 BY FOUR CAREER GROUPS

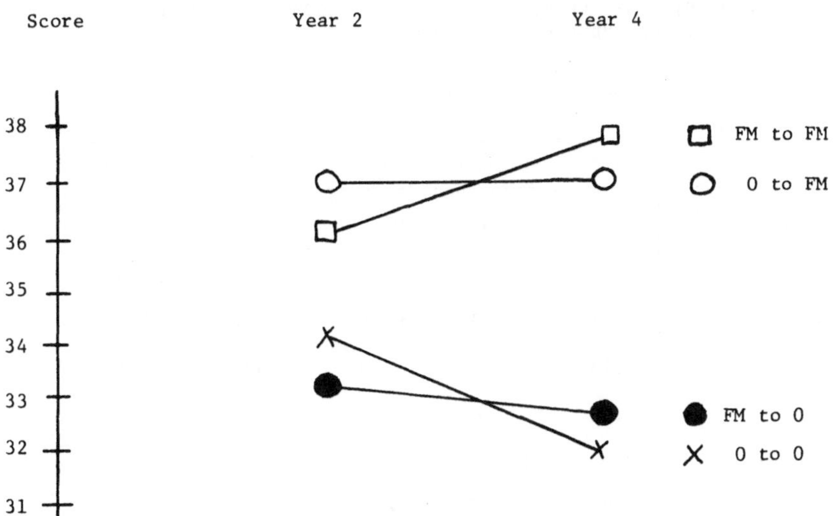

TABLE 3

A. PERCEPTIONS OF FAMILY MEDICINE AT YEAR 2 AND YEAR 4 BY STUDENTS MAINTAINING A COMMITMENT TO FAMILY MEDICINE THROUGHOUT MEDICAL SCHOOL

		Factor				
		Care	Science	Cure	Status	Outside
Year Two	$\bar{X}$	42.35	32.97	37.23	29.23	36.64
	S	5.52	3.28	4.70	4.95	6.67
Year Four	$\bar{X}$	39.91	35.31	36.41	29.69	38.75
	S	2.53	4.46	4.18	7.18	6.19
t		1.56	-1.63	.50	-.203	-.894
df		30	30	30	30	30
p		NS	NS	NS	NS	NS

B. PERCEPTIONS OF FAMILY MEDICINE AT YEAR 2 AND YEAR 4 BY STUDENTS CHOOSING SPECIALITIES OTHER THAN FAMILY MEDICINE THROUGHOUT MEDICAL SCHOOL

		Factor				
		Care	Science	Cure	Status	Outside
Year Two	$\bar{X}$	43.33	34.65	38.70	33.82	38.05
	S	4.41	5.99	3.64	7.07	9.37
Year Four	$\bar{X}$	39.52	30.83	34.58	34.17	30.00
	S	3.18	6.25	5.20	6.34	9.53
t		2.32	1.46	2.16	-.12	2.00
df		22	22	22	22	22
p		$p<.05$	NS	$p<.05$	NS	$p<.05$

The next data examined explore the changes which take place in the perception of family medicine by medical students, particularly by those who switched from family medicine to another specialty during the course of their medical school training. Table 4 and Figure 3 report mean perceptions of

Figure 2

A. PERCEPTIONS OF FAMILY MEDICINE BY FAMILY MEDICINE-FAMILY MEDICINE GROUP

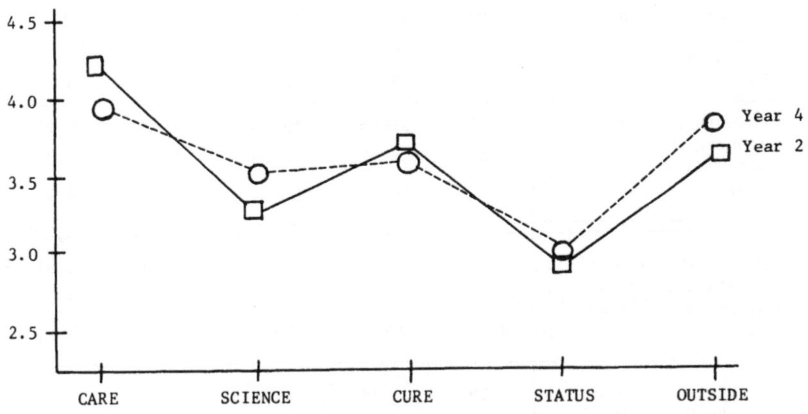

B. PERCEPTIONS OF FAMILY MEDICINE BY OTHER-OTHER GROUP

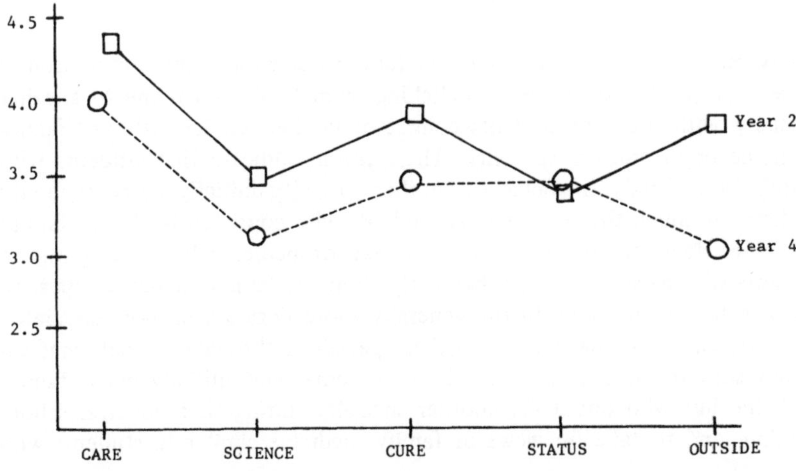

TABLE 4

A. YEAR 2 PERCEPTIONS

		Factor				
		Care	Science	Cure	Status	Outside
Students Always Choosing Family Medicine (FM-FM)	$\overline{X}$	42.35	32.97	37.23	29.23	36.64
	S	5.52	3.28	4.70	4.95	6.67
	N	16	16	16	16	16
Students Switching From Family Medicine to Other Specialties (FM-O)	$\overline{X}$	43.08	32.31	35.38	29.23	33.85
	S	4.08	6.96	7.06	7.32	10.44
	N	13	13	13	13	13
Students Always Choosing Other Specialties (O-O)	$\overline{X}$	43.33	34.65	38.70	33.82	38.05
	S	4.41	5.99	3.64	7.07	9.37
	N	12	12	12	12	12
Results of Two-Sample t-Tests Comparing (FM-FM) and (FM-O)	t	-.38	.33	.81	.00	.84
	df	27	27	27	27	27
	p	NS	NS	NS	NS	NS
Results of Two-Sample t-Tests Comparing (FM-O) and (O-O)	t	-.39	-.86	-1.40	-1.52	-1.01
	df	23	23	23	23	23
	p	NS	NS	NS	NS	NS

family medicine at year two and year four. These data permit comparison of these perceptions for students switching from family medicine to another specialty with those of students consistent in their choice either of family medicine or of another specialty. These results indicate that students who switch from family medicine to another specialty initially perceive family medicine in much the same way as students who consistently choose family medicine. However, by the end of four years of medical school, this group of students who have abandoned their early choice of family medicine appear to perceive family medicine in the generally more negative fashion associated with students who have chosen other specialties throughout their medical school sojourn. It appears that those students who initially chose family medicine but who opted for another specialty during their medical school training tend to take on views of family medicine similar to students who have always chosen other specialties; as time progresses they adopt views in which family medicine is seen less favorably.

As mentioned earlier, only four students represent the option of starting out with a choice of one of the specialties and switching to family medicine by the end of the fourth year. Although omitted from the tables and figures because of their small number, their scores at the end of the second year resemble those who consistently chose other specialties; however, at the end of the fourth year, they approximate the pattern of those who consistently chose family medicine. When looking at Table 4 and Figure 3 one can observe that for all students the scores for care drop from the second to the fourth year. The same can be said for the scores for cure even though for this factor those who choose family medicine at the end of the fourth year perceive family medicine higher in the factor cure than the other two groups. The scores for the science factor begs for further study, with the data suggesting

TABLE 4 (continued)

B. YEAR 4 PERCEPTIONS

		Factor				
		Care	Science	Cure	Status	Outside
Students Always Choosing Family Medicine (FM-FM)	$\bar{X}$	39.91	35.31	36.41	29.69	38.75
	S	2.53	4.46	4.18	7.18	6.19
	N	16	16	16	16	16
Students Switching From Family Medicine to Other Specialties (FM-O)	$\bar{X}$	38.35	29.81	32.69	28.85	31.54
	S	3.63	8.19	4.50	7.68	9.87
	N	13	13	13	13	13
Students Always Choosing Other Specialties (O-O)	$\bar{X}$	39.52	30.83	34.58	34.17	30.00
	S	3.18	6.25	5.20	6.34	9.53
	N	12	12	12	12	12
Results of Two-Sample t-Tests Comparing (FM-FM) and (FM-O)	t	1.31	2.22	2.23	0.29	2.31
	df	27	27	27	27	27
	p	NS	$p<.05$	$p<.05$	NS	$p<.05$
Results of Two-Sample t-Tests Comparing (FM-O) and (O-O)	t	-0.82	-1.02	-0.94	-1.80	0.38
	df	23	23	23	23	23
	p	NS	NS	NS	NS	NS

Figure 3

A. PERCEPTIONS OF FAMILY MEDICINE AT YEAR 2

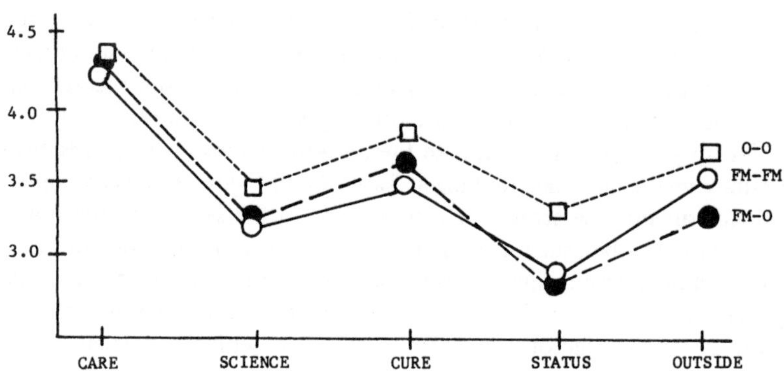

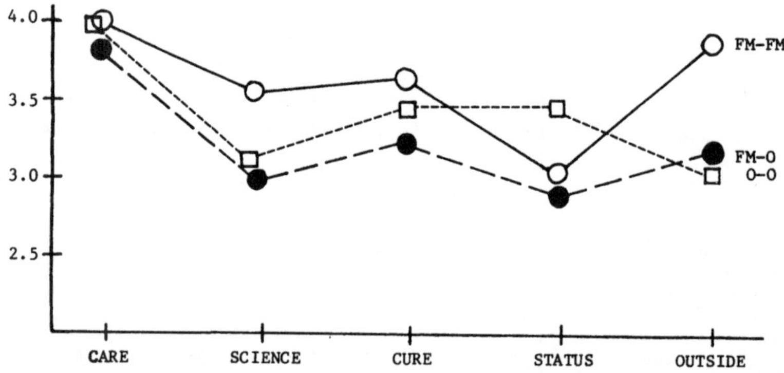

that at year four those who choose family medicine have noticeably increased their perception of the science component in family medicine while the two groups finally opting for other specialties associate less science with family medicine than they did 3 years earlier.

An examination of these data sets the stage for raising questions about the medical school experience and the recruitment and training of future family physicians. If borne out by further data, it appears that the basis for feeding the family medicine labor force depends on the recruitment of medical students who have already an interest in family medicine. Furthermore, the success of this recruitment process seems linked to self-defining qualities of medical students which may permit prediction of the persistence of early choices. The data reported here suggest that such a differentiating variable might be associated with a personal commitment to a "caring" orientation. It may be even more important to gain a better understanding of the factors which appear to make the medical school experience an environment which moves students away from chosing family medicine.

Medical School Environment

The medical students who were subjects of the study were interviewed twice during their clinical years, once before and once after a selected clinical block. These interviews yield a picture of values, pressures, rewards, and sanctions which suggest an environment in which the choice of family medicine can only be interpreted as a process of resistance against the dominant school culture. This statement is made notwithstanding the above reported fact, that the official school policy had expressed itself as being in full support of primary care and family medicine.

It is important for those committed to family medicine to examine the assumption that the medical school is a biased socializing environment and that its encounters and experiences mitigate against choosing family medicine as a career. It is equally important to acknowledge that this condition, if verified, does not suggest a conspiracy but rather a result of the very nature of the structure of modern medicine, its successes, and its impact on the social organization on the delivery of acute care. The structure and process of the medical curriculum reflect to a greater degree than medical educators have generally acknowledged the peculiarities of the university medical center which is, in most instances, an institution dedicated to tertiary medical care.

Science, Technology, and Multiple Specialties

The very successes in science and in technology achieved by modern medicine are deeply rooted in the social structure of the university medical environment. The dramatic accomplishments and the breakthroughs in diagnosis and in therapy have resulted in an evergrowing array of subspecialization and the emergence of dependence on an evergrowing number of specialized personnel within medicine or from newly developed specialty occupations. Relatively little attention has been paid in the literature to the consequence of this network of consulting subspecialties and technological instrumentation. While these achievements have enhanced the system's capability to diagnose and treat, they have created an environment which tends to diminish the experience of rewarding personal accountability and responsibility on the part of the physician.

Indeed, excellence in the practice of medicine is associated with the physician's use of multiple techniques of instrumentation and modes of obtaining laboratory data. As a corollary to the continuing myth of individualized medical practice looms the evidence of the emergence of a network of interdependence, diminishing individual responsibility, and the spreading of responsibility from one practitioner to a network of medical functionaries and to complex units of hardware. For every decision to be made, there are specialists whose judgment serves as a database or as backup and there are tests which are used to rule out other possibilities thus confirming by exclusion, if not by evidence. Dependence on using these resources is experienced by medical students as a desirable and rewarded mode of practice. The physician's decision becomes the summation of an array of data and diverse judgments. In a profound and possibly shocking sense, the socialization of the physician in the modern medical school may reflect a shift towards the development of a highly skilled and powerful technologist. This occurs at the expense of grooming a professional practitioner in the traditional sense of professional practice which, at least as reflected in past literature, has been synonymous with personal responsibility for professional behavior and personal accountability for client welfare (Goode, 1960).

If indeed the organizational reality of medical care and medical education reflects subspecialization and technological dependence, family medicine may represent structurally and symbolically a discordant note in the overall theme. Family medicine may indeed be a reaction to these subspecializing forces and may represent an attempt by some physicians to redefine and recapture an integrative role in the monitoring of health processes. If family medicine represents a reaffirmation of personal and professional accountability, then it is not surprising that the real experiences as the student passes through medical school make family medicine a less attractive choice by virtue of the nature of the medical role as observed and experienced during the third and fourth years.

Status and Rewards

This integrative stance taken by family medicine flies in the face of another fundamental component of American professional value structure. Modern Western society, particularly American society, is steeped in a tradition in which status and rewards are positively associated with degrees of specialization and with the precision by which boundaries of competence can be defined and defended. To "know more and more about less and less" is prestigious, and professional status seems to be negatively correlated with the size of the territory claimed as professional turf. Subspecialization also seems associated with complex requirements of formal training and demonstration of competence. Within this setting subspecialties, no matter how esoteric or infrequently called upon, are more likely to receive rewards and recognition than a field which by the very nature of its claims synthesizes rather than reduces, integrates rather than subdivides, and which chooses comprehensiveness and continuity as its criterion of expertise. Neither of these two dimensions can be defined easily by either territory or technology.

In an environment made up of a competitive and sometimes reluctant federation of medical subspecialists, family medicine can be expected to appear as a second class choice to students. The empowering flavor of subspecialty qualifications is reflected in Lewy's (1977, p. 879) account of general practitioners' reference to "those only trained in family medicine as 'medical eunuchs.'" The low status of the generalist is reflected in the study by Matteson and Smith (1977) which showed that medical students rank family medicine low in status within the medical profession.

Supporters of family medicine are frequently motivated by their concern with the need for physicians who are willing to practice in rural areas. One can observe a prevailing notion that a choice of family medicine is tantamount to a proclivity to select a rural practice site. Tables 5 and 6 show that by and large the tendency towards rural practice by those who choose family medicine results in only minor differences. What is interesting in these two tables is that the distribution of rural and urban origin and choices are consistent for both groups whose original specialty preference remained the same at the end of 4 years. Those who moved from an early choice of family medicine to opting for other specialties at the end of their medical education show a shift from rural origin to a choice of urban practice settings. Conversely the small number of medical students who moved to family medicine from initial preferences for other specialties appear to reflect a move from urban origin to a preference for rural practice. Here again the reporting of these initial data is only heuristic and suggestive because of the small numbers.

The Medical School as an Urban Setting

There is, however, another way in which the description of the social and professional world of the medical center is likely to influence the site of practice. Early in this paper it was suggested that specialization and division of labor with its ensuing fabric of functional interdependence and occupa-

TABLE 5

URBAN/RURAL ORIGIN BY FAMILY/OTHER CHOICE

	F→F	F→O	O→F	O→O	Total
Urban	8	4	4	8	24
Rural	7	8	0	4	19
	n=15	n=12	n=4	n=12	n=43

tional heterogeneity characterizes the medical center. The modern medical center is reminiscent of Wirth's traditional definition of urbanism (1938) which identified urbanism with density, permanence, heterogeneity, and specialization. As a community it is characterized by the high density of its population. Like in all urban settings conditions of high density give rise to impersonal, functionally specific relationships in which personal consideration and feelings give way to exchange of tasks and to interactions based on stereotypes. An urban setting sets the stage for a highly developed devision of labor with increasingly defensive concerns for territorial boundaries. The coordinator rather than the performer of primary tasks emerges as wielder of influence in the anonymous scene of the urban marketplace. Security stems from competence in increasingly circumscribed spheres and in protecting oneself from personal involvement with the multitude of face-to-face contacts (Simmel, 1936).

The medical school is indeed an urban institution and it rewards accommodation to urban ways of life. The medical center as it embraces the future physician rewards those medical students who fit well into a network of practice composed of a plethora of different specialties within medicine and involving a large number of other occupations; it rewards behavior which accommodates and conforms to the highly specialized performance of specified detailed tasks which result in a sequence of almost anonymously assembled processes. It rewards the learning of skills which enable the future physican to select data from a variety of laboratories and technologies and to translate them into diagnostic or therapeutic activities. In other words, within the framework of the current medical center, the future physician learns that quality of medical care is highly associated with the dependence on a large number of specialized skills, types of equipment, professional specialties, and the ability of collecting data from various sources as a prelude to medical decision-making.

Using the term socialization in describing the medical school experience implies that the encounters and events of these 4 years will not only teach content but will form personal and social identities and will also formulate habits, expectations, and a sense of comfort or discomfort in various professional settings. If the close proximity and dependence on resource personnel and technology becomes an index of security and quality, a choice of an urban practice setting and of a clearly defined specialty is more likely in the offing.

Thus far this paper has examined the medical school environment in terms of its structural and professional aspects. The curriculum itself provides not only subject matter, content, and practice experience but it also signals the real rather than the professed priorities of the system. As Becker et al. (1961) emphasized in their classic study, medical students, like all occupants of high pressure environments, learn early to distinguish between the language and the reality of the powers which control their fates. In most medical curricula the structure of the first 2 years emphasizes the primacy of the laboratory sciences and sets the stage for the prestige and reward structure of subspecialty competence. Courses devoted to "being a physician," whether couched as learning about taking histories, interviewing, or other aspects of the physician-patient contact, are generally of low prestige and considered the soft part of the first 2 years. In those few medical schools in which the behavioral sciences make an appearance in the first 2 years of the medical

TABLE 6

URBAN/RURAL CHOICE BY FAMILY/OTHER CHOICE

	F→F	F→O	O→F	O→O	Total
Urban	10	9	1	8	28
Rural	6	4	3	4	17
	n=16	n=13	n=4	n=12	n=45

curriculum, they are rarely valued, taken seriously, or perceived to represent a valid scientific or professional basis for the practice of medicine. What implication does this value pattern have for a specialty which claims comprehensiveness and response to patient experience as one axis of expertise?

The third and fourth year of the traditional medical school curriculum represents a different scenario. Typically, it is structured as a sequence of assignments to departmental domains. These are spheres of control and influence through which students pass on their way through required and elective territories. The clinical years belie the goal of a consistent integrated theme governing the educational processes of becoming a physician. On the contrary, the quasi-proprietary aura and the ethnocentrism and evangelism of various subfields of medicine make the student appear in some ways like a potential customer moving from sales exhibit to sales exhibit rather than as a future professional who, at all times, is enveloped in a climate of inquiry, relativity of knowledge, and invitations to raise new questions and to show intellectual skepticism.

The structure of the curriculum during the clinical years gives the impression of a topography with terrain features which range from those clearly visible and marked, to some which are barely identifiable. The traditional major specialties in medicine are clearly visible landmarks through which the student must pass as he travels through the curriculum. As Goode (1957, p. 196) observed, most professional programs "almost isolate their recruits from important lay contacts (and) furnish new ego ideals and reference groups." Some career options in medicine appear as optional places to visit during the third and fourth year while others are either not available or require special arrangements. Family medicine, a relatively recent arrival on the specialty scene, appears in different ways in different medical schools. Only rarely, however, is it a regular, required experience for all students. Lacking the structural reality of claimed time and space constitutes a message as far as student experience and student perceptions are concerned as long as allocation of student time in the third and fourth year curriculum reflects prestige and power among medical specialties, family medicine will not fare competitively in its bid for student choices.

The House Staff

Many of the observations offered in this paper have in one form or another been made by medical educators or researchers as part of a variety of commentaries about medical education. Thus, as these themes emerge from interviews they blend quickly into observations and data previously acquired by the authors. One finding emerged, however, which has not been addressed in the literature. The peculiar, powerful role of interns and residents in the education of medical students within a medical center appears to be so crucial in the process of career choice that it seems surprising that not more attention has been paid to this issue.

The problematic and ambiguous structural position of the house staff has been studied (Miller, 1970; Mumford, 1970) primarily as it affects their own career in the profession and as it influences patient care. While the period of residency is considered primarily to be a vehicle for postgraduate education, it is generally acknowledged that the house staff provides the bulk of medical practice in a large teaching hospital. In doing so, the house staff is the primary contact for medical students and thus also does most of the teaching. A large proportion of the teaching which takes place during the daily rounds involves the medical students with the residents and interns, frequently without the attending physician present. Sheer numbers, hours on the patient care unit, and informal gatherings cast the house staff as the medical students' dominant medical environment. The reports of the students interviewed testify to the fact that by far the largest amount of educational contact with practicing physicians occurred with house staff rather than with the faculty. It is from house staff that students report to have received not only educational content but also the climate and the culture of their block. The interviews suggest that the recruitment process into specialties emanates frequently from the interns and the residents rather than from the attending physician.

This insertion of interns and residents into the organizational structure and educational experience of the medical student has important consequences which are linked to the ambiguous social status of the house staff itself. They represent a classical example of a social category which, although placed into an acknowledged niche, remains, to a degree, structurally segregated from the institution in which they function. In some ways they are reminiscent of the classic description of the stranger (Simmel, 1952) who partakes in the activities of the group albeit continuously at the margin and who is neither incorporated into a socio-psychological group identity nor encumbered with the expectations of conforming completely to the group norms. As members of the house staff, interns and residents have loyalty to their specialty and to their department but are neither structurally nor socio-psychologically committed to the policies and philosophies evolved by the faculty and administration of the school of medicine. Thus, in a school of medicine in which academic administration and faculty assemblies have made a commitment to family medicine, this commitment and its underlying philosophy has no meaningful provisions for being transmitted to the house staff whose teaching roles are only minimally formalized, although shown to be a major educational reality. Values of their respective departments rather than the policies of the school will mingle with the orientations imported from their own respective former educational environments. Yet interns and residents serve as possibly one of the most influential shaping forces in the career choices and socialization experiences of future physicians.

Concluding Remarks

In this paper the point is made that the modern, complex medical center is not a favorable environment in which to develop a career commitment to the practice of family medicine. It has also been suggested that the apparent relative success of bringing new cohorts of young physicians into family medicine may be related to early, pre-medical school choices and that those who move into family medicine are the survivors of a larger, initial body of students oriented toward this version of primary care. The data in this paper report the tentative findings that those whose commitment to family medicine persists may bring a perception of themselves as "caring" professionals into the specializing environment of the medical center. The main thrust of this paper, however, is to emphasize that the specialty-favoring, urbanizing climate of the medical school is deeply embedded in the very nature of current medical science, its technology, and the social structure of patient care delivery.

With all the successes which family medicine has achieved since its inception it is still considered a problematic entity among medical specialties. Among the choices which this body of medical practitioners is forced to make are those which affect the recruitment of students into this specialty. This question may, however, be not merely one of assuring numbers. A more important issue, as suggested in this paper, may be the kind of novice who is attracted to family medicine as its image, its message, and its reality may undergo changes. One could oversimplify the implications of this paper as suggesting that those attributes of family medicine which currently seem to attract recruits are the very ones which account for this specialty's low status and influence. Acquiring the claims to traditional academic medical respectability may gain territory for family medicine at the expense of attracting those to whom family medicine represents, at this time, the way of being a physician. The question to be addressed in the future involves the issue of the quality and characteristics of students attracted or lost as family medicine maintains or alters its image and structure.

Family medicine seems confronted on one hand by the academic values of medical laboratory science, demonstrable territorial and functional claims, and control over unique technologies. On the other hand, family medicine symbolizes comprehensive primary care with romantic overtones of a return to the good old days of the personal physician. While there is reality to this dichotomy, a third model with its own opportunities and dangers can be identified in the dialogue governing the future of family medicine.

If the name of the specialty and the justifications given for its emergence are taken literally, family medicine can be seen as the specialty which translates the comprehensive experience of illness and the striving for health into a systematic body of expertise using the context of family life as the basis for research and practice. If the links between family process, personal existence, and organismic functions become the basis of scientific expertise (Mauksch, 1974), family medicine can claim a territory, a domain of research, and a field of preeminent practice. At the same time this field of competence is based on the human service demands and takes its justification from the needs for personal care and continuity. Thus, it would seem that family medicine could simultaneously capture academic respectability and symbolic appeal. Yet this option, as appealing as it may be, forces family medicine far afield from the traditional primary reliance on the biological and physical sciences and forces a link of family medicine with the social sciences which, at best, are suspect and untested as a scientific basis for the practice of medicine. Regardless of its scientific and philosophic merit, the politics of embracing the social sciences are risky. The full development of this model may involve early struggles but may, in the long run, provide family medicine a defined place in the sun and a significant contribution to the health care needs of our society.

REFERENCES

Becker, H. S., Geer, B. Hughes, E. C., & Strauss, A. L. *Boys in white: Student culture in a medical school.* Chicago: University of Chicago Press, 1961.

Brent, E. Criteria for medical student choices. Unpublished draft, University of Missouri-Columbia, 1977.

Cullison, S., Reid, J. C., & Colwill, J. M. Medical school admissions, specialty selections, and distribution of physicians. *Journal of the American Medical Association*, 1976, *235*, 502-505.

Goode, W. J. Community Within a Community: The Professions. *American Sociological Review*, 1957, *22*, 194-200.

Goode, W. J. Encroachment, charlatanism, and the emerging profession: Psychology, medicine and sociology. *American Sociological Review*, 1960, *25*, 902-914.

Harman, H. *Modern factor analysis*. Chicago: University of Chicago Press, 1960.

Lewy, R. M. The emergence of the family practitioner: An historical analysis of a new specialty. *Journal of Medical Education*, 1977, *52*, 873-881.

Liccione, W. J., & McAllister, S. Attitudes of first year medical students toward rural medical practice. *Journal of Medical Education*, 1974, *49*, 449-451.

Matteson, M. T., & Smith, S. V. Medical specialty choice: A note on status ranking. *Social Science and Medicine*, 1977, *11*, 421-423.

Mauksch, H. O. A social science basis for conceptualizing family health. *Social Science and Medicine*, 1974, *8*, 521-528.

Mauksch, H. O. The nurse: A study in role perception. Unpublished doctoral dissertation, University of Chicago, 1960.
Miller, S. J. *Prescription for leadership: Training for the medical elite*. Chicago: Aldine Publishing, 1970.

EDUCATION FOR THE PRACTICE OF FAMILY MEDICINE

John P. Geyman, MD

The voice of the public has become more audible in recent years concerning availability, adequacy, and cost of health care. The consumer has become more disenchanted each year with the high cost and fragmentation of health care services. Most families have many physicians, none of whom has a comprehensive picture of their health status. Primary care is often not readily available, and the pressure on hospital emergency rooms has become intense. There is considerable evidence that the public still desires a family doctor (Marchmont-Robinson, Note 1).

The Millis, Willard, and Folsom reports of 1966 (Notes 2-4), followed in 1969 by the recognition by the American Medical Association of family practice as our 20th specialty, have led to a major reorientation of medical education in the United States. In the last 10 years we have seen the rapid development of new educational programs in family medicine at all levels. This paper will attempt to provide an overview of the philosophy, goals, content, and initial directions of these educational programs which relate directly to the future role of the practicing family physician in this country.

Renaissance of Interest

That there is a true renaissance of interest in family practice in recent years cannot be denied. Perhaps the most obvious measure of this new interest can be seen in today's medical students. A common story in many medical schools, particularly in the last several years, is that up to one-quarter or one-third of each class is seriously considering family practice as a career.

A large proportion of current medical students show a serious concern for the present inequities between the potential for health care and the actual quality and quantity of health care delivered to the population. Students are becoming more interested in social and community problems as they relate to

Dr. Geyman is Professor and Chairman, Department of Family Medicine, University of Washington, Seattle, WA 98195.

medical care. Many are reacting against the extent of specialization in the traditional medical school experience and are more interested in a holistic approach to patient care. The burden is now on the medical schools to respond to the critical need for more family physicians and to develop quality training programs which will attract sufficient students into this field.

In the 11 years since family practice was recognized as a specialty, divisions or departments of family practice have been started in over three-quarters of the nation's medical schools. There is a concurrent "loosening up" of undergraduate medical education. Many of the current trends in medical schools favor the development of family practice as a specialty, including the following:

1. Contracting a proportion of undergraduate medical education devoted to basic sciences with a closer definition of those portions of each basic science which are clinically relevant.
2. Earlier clinical exposure to patients.
3. Increased proportion of elective time.
4. Larger classes, which necessitate considerable decentralization of clinical training.
5. Greater use of preceptorships with practicing physicians and clerkships in outlying community hospitals.
6. Increasing emphasis on ambulatory care, health care delivery, and community medicine.

Curricular revisions in many medical schools in response to these trends afford medical students increased opportunities to become involved with a variety of learning experiences in family practice settings both within the school and in the community.

In addition, there are powerful trends outside of medical schools themselves which are exerting strong pressure in favor of family practice. Among these trends are the following:

1. A growing void in the number of physicians trained and interested in primary care.
2. Increased fragmentation and depersonalization of health care through increased specialization and overbureaucratization of medical and health care systems.
3. Increased cost of inefficient and uncoordinated health care services.
4. Increased emphasis on accessibility and comprehensiveness of health care for a growing population.

5. Growing importance of consumer input to health planning and policy issues.

Stephens suggests that the modern rise of family practice education cannot be understood without recognizing the historical concept of reform. In his words: "The medical establishment itself is created to a considerable degree by forces that originate in the larger social order–forces of political, economic and cultural significance for society as a whole. It is my belief that family practice education bears a special, perhaps even a unique relation to these external forces, and that its current significance and future development lie in our understanding of these forces and relationships" (Stephens, Note 5).

There has been considerable legislative support of family practice in the last several years. Departments of family practice in state medical schools have been legislated in New Jersey, New York, Illinois, Kentucky, and North Carolina. Other state legislatures, such as Nebraska, Minnesota, South Carolina, and Virginia, have appropriated substantial funds to their medical schools earmarked for family practice. At the federal level, we have likewise seen considerable funding allocated to developing family practice programs.

Some Basic Definitions

It is useful to start with some basic definitions before discussing educational programs.

The "family," as the basic unit of care in family practice, is defined more broadly than the traditional nuclear family. Ransom and Vandervoort (Note 6) have defined the family as "a significant group of intimates, with a history and a future." Smilkstein (Note 7) has defined the family as "adult partners, with or without children, and single parents with children. These people function in a setting where there is a sense of home and they have an agreement to establish nurturing relationships.

The "family physician" has been defined by The American Academy of Family Physicians as a physician who (Note 8):

1. Serves as the physician of first contact and provides an accessible means of entry into the health care system.
2. Evaluates his/her patients' total health needs, provides personal health care within his range of competency, and refers patients when indicated to other specialists or community resources.
3. Accepts responsibility for his/her patients' total health care, including the use of consultants, within the context of the family and community.

4. Acts as a coordinator of his/her patients' health services.

The family physician can thus be viewed as a specialist in breadth, using multiple disciplines and providing primary, continuing, and comprehensive health care to all members of the family, regardless of age, sex, or presenting complaint.

"Family practice," as the name of the new specialty, denotes the process of application of the knowledge and skills of the family physician as he/she delivers health care to families.

Family medicine is the academic discipline which is acquired and applied by the family physician (Geyman, Note 9). This discipline can be satisfactorily defined as that body of knowledge and skills applied by the family physician as he/she provides primary, continuing, and comprehensive health care to patients and their families. It is a horizontal discipline, sharing portions of all other clinical disciplines from which it is derived but applying to families such derivative portions in a unique and holistic way. In addition, family medicine includes new, incompletely developed components, such as family dynamics in health and disease and its own areas of research. Family medicine is, therefore, the only field in medicine which directs itself primarily to the total health needs of the patient and his/her family, with emphasis on the integration of health services with the least degree of fragmentation.

The discipline of family medicine can be further described as: (a) including an area of competency to deal with well over 90% of all health problems of the family*; (b) involving the responsibility to arrange and coordinate referral to other specialists and community resources when indicated; (c) including responsibility for patient care both in and out of the hospital, with emphasis on more effective ambulatory care; and (d) requiring teamwork with an expanding health team.

"Primary care" is a term which has been the subject of considerable confusion and varied definitions in recent years. Although it is beyond the scope of this paper to explore this issue in depth, each of several definitions includes several elements: first contact care, comprehensiveness, and continuity of care, and coordination of care through utilization of consultants and community resources. The object of primary care involves some basic differences. Thus, the family physician is the primary care physician for the family and for patients of all ages and both sexes; the general internist may serve as a primary care physician for adults; the general pediatrician may act as a

---

*Two recent studies of referral patterns of family physicians have shown that only 2% to 3% of patient visits involve referral to other consultants (Metcalfe & Sischy, Note 10), (Geyman et al., Note 11).

primary care physician for children; and the obstetrician-gynecologist may serve as a primary care physician (in a more limited way) for women.

Undergraduate Level

We are seeing active development of undergraduate programs in family medicine in a majority of the medical schools in this country. Under the direction of divisions or departments of family medicine, elective and core courses are being offered at various levels of undergraduate training (Note 12). One such curriculum in family practice has been well described by Barnett (Note 13). Although the goals of these programs will vary somewhat among institutions, the following are typical goals which are common to most programs:

1. To provide exposure to the content and orientation of family practice in contrast to other clinical specialties.
2. To illustrate the process of family practice through role models of exemplary family physicians.
3. To increase understanding of the stages of primary care–health maintenance, early diagnosis of asymptomatic disease, care of acute and chronic illness, rehabilitation, and care of terminal illness.
4. To increase understanding of the family as a unit in health and illness.
5. To consider the environmental, psychosocial, and socioeconomic determinants of disease and measures which can be taken by the physician to ameliorate these factors.
6. To help the student acquire problem-solving skills in the diagnosis and management of common clinical problems.
7. To provide an introduction of methodology of patient care audit and research in primary care.

Family practice contributes to undergraduate medical education in such areas as clinical correlation with the basic sciences, patient interviewing, physicial diagnosis, family dynamics, preventive medicine, and related areas. A variety of learning settings are used at the university base, in affiliated community hospitals, and in the offices of practicing family physicians. In the short span of the last several years, it has already been demonstrated that these programs effectively build and maintain considerable student interest in family practice as a career. For example, state medical schools with departments of family practice recently reported an average of 25% of their graduates opting for further training in family practice. Fifty-five percent of the graduates of one medical school have entered family practice residencies (Note 14).

Graduate Level

It is impressive how much progress has been made during the last 10 years in the development of graduate training programs in family practice. There are now over 370 approved family practice residency programs in the United States with over 6,000 residents in training. These are 3-year residency programs which prepare their graduates for certification by the American Board of Family Practice. Although the majority of these programs are based in community hospitals, many programs are being developed in the universities, and there is an increasing trend toward university affiliations with community hospitals. Competition among medical students is intense for family practice residency positions and the "fill rate" is high.

The curriculum of any family practice residency program in an integrated manner helps each resident to meet four major goals: (1) required breadth of knowledge, (2) required breadth of skills, (3) appropriate attitudes, and (4) habits of self-evaluation and continuing education.

The overall goal of residency training is to produce well-trained family physicians with several attributes:

1. Excellence as clinicians capable of providing definitive care of over 90% of health problems of individuals and their families.
2. Skill in each of the five stages of comprehensive health care: (a) prevention; (b) early diagnosis of asymptomatic disease; (c) emergency care, management of acute and chronic disease; (d) rehabilitation; and (e) management of incurable and terminal disease.
3. Understanding of own limitations, with ability to relate appropriately to consultants and other community resources.
4. Knowledge and sensitivity to behavioral aspects of health and illness for families, with capacity to recognize, and often manage, common behavioral disorders.
5. Attitudes which facilitate constructive relationships with patients, peers, consultants, and other members of the health care team and which also allow for sharing of responsibility for patient care in a group setting.

Family practice residencies stress continuity of care on a family basis. Residents care for an increasing number of families during their 3 years in residency. Their principal base is the model family practice unit (Family Practice Center), which approximates the office of a practicing family physician. Additional training is provided through clinical rotations on hospital services, specialty clinics, preceptorships, and elective experiences. The breadth of training in a family practice residency is unequaled by any other residency program. Training is provided in internal medicine, pediatrics, obstetrics-gynecology, minor surgery, behavioral science, preventive medicine, emergency care, and appropriate parts of numerous subspecialties such as cardiology, dermatology, otolaryngology, orthopedics, urology, and others. Particular attention is directed to the integration of behavioral science with clinical medicine through a process which has been well described by McWhinney (Note 15) and Bauman and Grace (Note 16).

The family practice residency program is directed toward three distinct capability levels:

1. Definitive capability (including, for example, the management of most common clinical and behavioral problems of families and life-threatening emergencies).
2. Partial capability (including the initiation of appropriate diagnostic and/or therapeutic measures for more complex clinical problems requiring consultation and/or referral).
3. Limited capability (including the recognition or suspicion of rare or complex clinical problems for referral).

This concept forms a rational foundation for a residency's curriculum which gives maximal emphasis to the knowledge and skills required for definitive capability. Lesser emphasis is given to the other two functional categories; in these areas, residents learn their particular limitations as well as how to best utilize consultation and referral to other specialists and community resources.

Postgraduate Level

Continuing medical education at the postgraduate level is now recognized as a critical requirement for the maintenance of clinical competence in all fields. It has been estimated that 75% or more of a physician's entire medical education over a practice career will be on the postgraduate level (Farber, Note 17). The Willard report has stated that "with the half-life of total medical information estimated at something less than five years, it is no longer possible for any physician to depend on the quality of his undergraduate medical education, internship, and residency to sustain him at a level of professional excellence throughout his career" (Note 18).

Family practice is the first specialty in American medicine to establish required recertification. Diplomates of the American Board of Family Practice will be reexamined every 6 years by examination and by audit of their hospital and office records.

With the increased importance of continuing education in family practice, we are seeing new emphasis on several new approaches.

1. Increased emphasis on small-group teaching and self-instructional approaches rather than the lecture method.
2. Profiling of individual physicians' practices (i.e., by kinds of clinical problems encountered, age and sex characteristics of practice, etc.) as an approach to help plan for specific educational needs.
3. Increasing use of the problem-oriented medical record* and audit of records.
4. Self-assessment examinations which can identify individual educational needs.
5. Increased opportunities for practicing family physicians to become involved with teaching programs on a part-time basis.
6. Consultation with other specialists as a teaching and learning process.

Discussion

Family medicine represents a new force in medical education and practice. This specialty is particularly concerned with such areas as continuity of care, incorporation of behavioral science into clinical practice, care of the family as a unit, health maintenance, team practice, audit, and self-assessment. Beyond the impact of these directions and the concurrent emphasis on ongoing personal care of individuals and their families, family medicine can be expected to contribute in an increasing way to our knowledge of common health problems in primary care, including the natural history of disease, its prevention, early diagnosis, and more effective management.

In the interrelated areas of patient care, education, and research, family practice must draw upon many disciplines in order to advance the discipline of family medicine. At the patient care level, for example, the family physician relates on a collegial and team basis with such disciplines as clinical pharmacology, psychology, medical sociology, social work, and various allied

*The problem-oriented medical record, first developed by Dr. Larry Weed (Note 19), bases the medical record on problems as encountered in practice, which are often less specific than actual disease entities (e.g., abdominal pain, marital problem, etc.).

health fields. Educational programs necessarily involve the important contributions of medical educators, behavioral scientists, and other disciplines involved in teaching in the setting of patient care. Research activities involve the collaboration of still other disciplines, such as epidemiology and biostatistics.

The future of family medicine rests, in largest measure, on the continued improvement of its educational programs; integration of new knowledge, skills, and techniques through research; and development of more effective approaches to the care of families. All of these efforts come together in evolving teaching programs as a continuum with three phases–graduate, graduate, and postgraduate. In the long run, the content, quality, and effectiveness of these educational programs will have a direct and specific bearing on several critical outcomes–recruitment of medical students for careers in family practice, adequacy of preparation of residency graduates for varied practice settings, identification and profile of the evolving specialty of family practice, and the capability of this field to meet growing deficits in primary care.

REFERENCE NOTES

1. Marchmont-Robinson, H. Today's challenge. *The Journal of the American Medical Association*, 1968, *204*, 247.

2. The graduate education of physicians. *The Report of the Citizens Commission of Graduate Medical Education*, 1966, Chicago: AMA.

3. Health is a community affair. *The Report of the National Commission on Community Health Services*, Cambridge: Harvard University Press, 1966.

4. Stephens, G. G. Reform in the United States: Its impact on medicine and education for family practice. *The Journal of Family Practice*, 1976, *3*(5), 507-512.

5. Ransom, D. C., & Vandervoort, H. E. The development of family medicine: Problematic trends. *The Journal of the American Medical Association*, 1973, *225*, 1098-1102.

6. Smilkstein, G. The family in trouble–How to tell. *The Journal of Family Practice*, 1975, *2*(1), 19-24.

7. Education for family practice. Prepared by Commission on Education, American Academy of General Practice, Kansas City, MO, August, 1969, 2-6.

8. Geyman, J. Family medicine as an academic discipline. *Journal of Medical Education*, 1971, *46*, 816.

9. Metcalfe, D. H. H., & Sischy, D. Patterns of referral from family practice. *The Journal of Family Practice*, 1974, *1*(2), 34-38.

10. Geyman, J. P., Brown, T. C., & Rivers, K. Referrals in family practice: A comparative study by geographic region and practice setting. *The Journal of Family Practice*, 1976, *3*(2), 163-167.

11. Leaman, T. L. Predoctoral education in family medicine: A ten-year perspective. *Journal of Family Practice*, 1979, *9*(5), 845-854.

12. Barnett, L. Carving an undergraduate curriculum in family practice. *The Journal of Family Practice*, 1974, *1*(3/4), 20-22.

13. Boulger, I. G. Family practice in the predoctoral curriculum: A model for success. *The Journal of Family Practice*, 1980, *10*(3), 453-458.

14. McWhinney, I. R. Beyond diagnosis–An approach to the integration of behavioral science and clinical medicine. *New England Journal of Medicine*, 1972, *287*(8), 384-387.

15. Bauman, M. H., & Grace, N. T. Family process and family practice. *The Journal of Family Practice*, 1974, *1*(2), 24-26.

16. Farber, S. In relevance today and tomorrow in medical education. *California Medicine*, 1970, *112*(69).

17. Meeting the challenge of family practice. *Report of the Ad Hoc Committee on Education for Family Practice of the Council on Medical Education*, Chicago: AMA, 1966, 28.

18. Weed, L. L. Medical records, medical education and patient care. Cleveland, OH: The Press of Case Western Reserve University, 1970.

THE COMPREHENSIVE FAMILY MEDICINE TRAINING PROGRAM: HAS SOCIOLOGY FOUND A PLACE IN GRADUATE MEDICAL EDUCATION?

Barbara Howe, PhD, JD
Perry S. Warren

The Mandate for a Sociologically-Oriented Physician

The idea that physical man reflects social man is not a new one in medicine, as medical historians such as Siegerist (1960), Shryock (1960), Haggard (1929), and Dubos (1959) will attest. Even with reference only to the post-Flexnerian era of scientific specialized medicine in the United States, the need is well established for physicians who are oriented to physical man as a social creature influenced by family and environment.

As early as 1942, for instance, proposals were made to the American Medical Association that the general practitioner be considered a specialist (Rardin, 1963, p. 153-163). The University of North Carolina was teaching a family physician's approach by 1956, including visits to patients' homes as part of the clinical experience (Fleming, 1956, p. 711-713). By 1960, the University of Vermont's Department of Preventive Medicine was assigning two local families to each third and fourth year medical student after an orientation that began with first year courses in human ecology (Haynes, 1960, p. 1340-1341).

Real headway in formalizing the concept and curriculum of family medicine was made in the 1960s. In 1962 the section on general practice of the AMA recognized a need for a specially trained physician who could manage comprehensive care of his patients (Rardin, 1962, p. 545-547) and in 1964 the American Board of General Practice for Family Physicians was incorporated (Walsh, 1970, p. 1192). Most importantly, several blue-ribbon commissions were formed to recommend solutions to a "crisis" in health care—a

Dr. Howe is Associate Professor, Department of Sociology, State University of New York at Buffalo, Buffalo, NY 14214. Mr. Warren is President, Institute for Health, 3300 East First Ave., Suite 340, Denver, CO 80206.

Marriage & Family Review, Vol. 4(1/2), Spring/Summer 1981

crisis which featured rising medical costs, manpower shortages, uneven distribution of care and fragmentation of the individual patient as he was treated by myriad clinical specialists. As John Walsh has noted:

> The year 1966 was a landmark in medical education circles when three significant reports were each independently reported and published: (1) *The Graduate Education of Physicians*, Report of the Citizen's Commission on Graduate Medical Education Commissioned by the AMA (Millis Commission Report); (2) *Health is a Community Affair*, Report of the National Commission on Community Health Services (Folsom Report); and (3) *Meeting the Challenge of Family Practice*, Report of the Ad Hoc Committee on Education for Family Practice of the AMA Council on Medical Education (Willard Report, 1970, p. 1193).

The reports of the Millis Commission (1966), the Willard Commission (1966), and the Folsom Commission (1966) held one important fact in agreement: medical education was in need of a change in orientation before the health needs of the nation could be met. To effect the goal of comprehensive health care a new type of specialist was going to be required. The Folsom Commission (1966) said:

> This physician should be aware of the many and varied social, emotional, and environmental factors that influence the health of his patient and his patient's family. He will either render or direct the patient to whatever services best suit his needs. His concern will be for the patient as a whole and his relationship with the patient must be a continuing one. In order to carry out his coordinating role, it is essential that all pertinent health information be channeled through him regardless of what institution, agency, or individual renders the service. He will have knowledge of the access to all health resources in the community–social, preventive, diagnostic, therapeutic, and rehabilitative–and will mobilize them for the patient.

An official call has been made by the Folsom Commission (1966) for the development of medical training programs that would produce physicians who could understand and treat each patient as a person whose health reflected and affected his roles in the family and community.

The Millis Report (1966) also recommended the training of physicians who could bring order to the specialized and fragmented field of medicine. The Ad Hoc Committee specified exactly what this new specialist should do:

> The family physician is one who: (1) serves as the physician of first contact with the patient and provides a means of entry into the health care system; (2) evaluates the patient's total health needs, provides personal medical care within one or more fields of medicine, and refers the patient when indicated to appropriate sources of care while preserving the continuity of his care; (3) assumes responsibility for the patient's comprehensive and continuous health care and acts as leader or coordinator of the team that provides health services; and (4) accepts the responsibility of the patient's total health care within the context of his environment, including the community and the family or comparable social unit (Willard Report, 1966, p. 7).

In its report the Ad Hoc Committee also recommended an eight point program for the medical education of family physicians. It was felt that the Committee's guidelines would help medical educators anticipate the future in preparing family physicians for a rapidly changing nation. The recommendations were: (1) the education program for family practice should take into account the changing character and content of higher education; (2) the family physician must be a complete physician learned in scientific medicine, and skilled in diagnosis and treatment; (3) in addition to scientific orientation, the family physician must be grounded in the behavioral sciences; (4) he must be exposed to research in educational methods, patient care, and distribution of medical services; (5) he must be allowed to practice and learn in a model of family practice; (6) the attitude and philosophy of all the medical school faculty must be supportive and constructive of family medicine; (7) family medicine must be recognized as a distinct entity within the educational institution and should be given the same status, budget, autonomy, etc.; and (8) the guidelines for family practice must be free and flexible. Rigid standardization would be senseless since heretofore there had been few models of successful training programs in family medicine (Willard Report, 1966, p. 15-16).

In addition to the eight-point program, the Committee suggested that the medical schools consider applicants with a broad range of interests and a broad range of undergraduate training (Willard Report, 1966, p. 17). They further emphasized the extreme importance of the behavioral and social sciences: "These disciplines (e.g., sociology, social psychology, and anthropology) should help the student acquire a holistic approach to health and disease and to recognize the interrelationships of cultural, social, psychological, and environmental factors with the psysiological and biochemical processes of the body" (Willard Report, 1966, p. 27).

Evaluation of the Mandate

The important potential role of sociology in the curriculum of the family physician programs has been endorsed repeatedly before, during, and since the publication of the above-mentioned blue-ribbon commission reports (Silver, 1963, p. 74-77; GP, 1966, p. 225-246; Harrell, 1970, p. 61-64). That potential role has been greatly enhanced by the passage of the Health Education and Manpower Act in 1976, which mandated that by 1980, 50% of all medical students graduating from medical school should be entering residencies in the three designated primary care specialties–internal medicine, pediatrics, and family practice. An additional aspect of this act was the allocation of some $40,000,000 for the expansion and improvement of existing family medicine residencies and for the creation of additional residency programs.

The question at hand–almost 12 years after these recommendations were submitted to medical educators–is whether a new breed of physicians is being produced by training in family medicine. Is there a new type of physician who is "aware not only of his patient's physicial illness, but also of interrelations of family members and of family and community and socioeconomic factors affecting the health of family members?" (Silver, 1965, p. 188-189).

There are clearly two elements that must be distinguished in evaluating this mandate to train family physicians–one quantitative and the other qualitative. As far as quantitative changes in the attention paid to training family physicians, there can be no doubt that significant shifts have occurred in the past decade. In 1967, there were only three family medicine training programs in the United States, at the Universities of Miami (Florida), Rochester, and Oklahoma. By 1970 there were 49 programs, in 1975 there were 233, and in 1977 there were well over 300.[1] In 1970 family practice became a board specialty, recognizing both general practitioners and new family practitioners who pass the specialty board examination.

It is clear that the combined availability of the many new residency programs in family medicine and the prestige available from board certifica-

---

[1]Data obtained from authors' communication with the American Academy of Family Physicians, May, 1975.

tion have increased the percent of medical students choosing family practice in the 1960s (Oates & Feldman, 1974, p. 562-569). Therefore, there has been a quantitative impact traceable to the 1960s recommendations to increase both the total supply of practicing physicians and the proportion becoming primary care physicians in particular. The most significant impetus to growth has been federal and state legislation requiring the development of primary care residencies and requiring medical students to enter them, and the large funding allocation from the federal government to expand and improve family medicine residencies and to begin pediatric and internal medicine residencies.

The qualitative changes in the type of training available in the new family practice programs have not been as well documented as the change in the quantity of family doctors. One question is the integration of any behavioral science perspective in family physician training, but from a sociological viewpoint it is also worth evaluating the place of sociology, in particular, within the behavioral science contribution. Twelve years after the three major commissions called for the integration of a sociological perspective into the training of family physicians, the question that must be addressed is whether substantial progress has been made in implementing sociology courses in family medicine training programs.

To evaluate the question of the status and impact of academic sociology in family medicine training in the United States, a survey of all 322 approved family practice training programs was made in late 1977, with a response rate of 82.9%. Of the 267 respondents, six stated that their program was just under development and they would not have residents until July of 1978. The remaining 261 respondents provided information on the age and size of their program and answered questions pertinent to the role of sociology and of behavioral science within the training programs. The survey's first question was: "Is sociology a part of the residents' curriculum?" This was followed by a definition: "Sociology is the scientific study of human group life and social behavior. Is that what you have?" One hundred eight stated that they did have sociology as part of their residents' curriculum. The second part of question was asked: "If yes, is there a sociology course?" The responses ranged over a wide spectrum. Most of the programs that did have sociology stated that they had it integrated into their entire behavioral science curriculum, which consisted of a variety of encounters with the physicians/residents. This included weekly seminars, grand rounds, didactic sessions, etc. No clear cut pattern of how the material was presented appeared.

The second question, "Is there a sociologist on your faculty?" received 53 positive responses. The second part of the question asked them to identify the training of the individuals who were described as sociologists. Of the 53 individuals cited, 35 had PhD's in sociology or social psychology, eight had master's degress in sociology, and three had bachelor's degrees. The remaining 17 had degrees in psychology, social work, and communications. The survey results here reiterate a problem addressed in our questionnaire design—the definition of sociology by nonsociologists. Even after indicating that they have sociology in their curriculum, for instance, only 50% answered yes to the question, "Is there a sociologist on the faculty?" However, of those 53 only 39 programs actually had faculty with sociological training at any degree level. This is not to say that other behavioral scientists are or are not equipped to present basic sociological concepts to family medicine residents. The point is that they are doing so. A summary of the responses is provided in Table 1 below.

Further analysis of these findings indicates that the integration of sociology into family practice curricula cannot be predicted from the age of a family practice training program.

The size of the family practice program is not related to the presence or absence of sociology in the curriculum. The size of the programs that did offer sociology in some form was only slightly larger than the mean size of all family practice programs.

Finally, on the question of the presence or absence of a sociologist on the medical faculty, again, size and age were not predictors. The most outstanding characteristic of those programs with a sociologist on the faculty was that they were present in those programs affiliated with major universities. In fact, it can be inferred that of those programs indicating they had a sociologist on the faculty, the sociologist's affiliation in each case was essentially with the university rather than with the family practice program.

Why has not sociology become an integral part of family medicine resi-

TABLE 1

INDICATORS OF SOCIOLOGY'S INTEGRATION IN FAMILY PRACTICE TRAINING PROGRAMS

	Is sociology a part of the FP resident's curriculum?	Is there a sociologist on the faculty?
YES	108	53
NO	153	208

TABLE 2

AGE OF FAMILY PRACTICE PROGRAMS AS RELATED TO INTEGRATION OF SOCIOLOGY INTO CURRICULUM

Mean age of all programs	4.21 years
Mean age of programs with sociology as part of curriculum either required or as an elective	4.25 years

TABLE 3

SIZE OF FAMILY PRACTICE PROGRAMS AS RELATED TO INTEGRATION OF SOCIOLOGY INTO CURRICULUM (SIZE MEASURED AS NUMBER OF RESIDENTS)

Mean size of all programs	18.24
Mean size of all programs with sociology in curriculum or course	18.65

dency programs in an era when the programs have proliferated and sociologists are underemployed? First, it appears that even the commissioners[2] who recommended the sociologically oriented family practice program did not know how a sociological perspective could be integrated into the medical training program. "It is not clear at this time," said the Ad Hoc Committee, "how best to incorporate the behavioral sciences in education for family practice" (Willard Report, 1966, p. 28). The Millis Commission agreed, saying that "It is not possible to be specific about content, organization, or degree of emphasis" of sociology input into the training of family physicians

[2]It should be noted that on the Ad Hoc, Folsom, and Coggeshall Commissions there were no sociologists; the Millis Commission had one, Everett C. Hughes.

because "there has not been sufficient experience with the teaching of the medical applications of these topics" (Millis Report, 1966, p. 51).

It appears also that the presentation of the core of a highly theoretical discipline to clinically oriented students cannot be done by the traditional didactic methods familiar to the academic sociologist. Some substantial efforts in this direction have been made; the reports of the conference series on behavioral sciences and medical education [DHEW Pub. No. (NIH) 72-41] is an example. Further questions arise concerning the organizational placement of behavioral sciences within university family medicine programs. What is needed are innovative teaching strategies so that any book-learned theoretical material becomes immediately relevant to the practicing resident. Whatever the specifics, it is suggested that if a sociological perspective is to be imparted to the clinician, it should not be done in an episodic or case-by-case approach; instead, the goal should be the training of a physician who sees his whole patient panel in the context of the family and community of which each is a member.

From the viewpoint of the many behavioral scientists who devoted the last decade or more to bringing a substantive behavioral science perspective into family medicine training programs, and even formally organizing themselves to do so in the Association of Behavioral Scientists in Medical Education, attention to disciplinary labeling among them may seem trivial or even counter-productive. Behavioral science as opposed to sociology, anthropology, or social work is the label which was being applied in family medicine training programs. The requirement for a more applied approach to educating family physicians has required the specific behavioral scientist to become a generalist, as the residency program has been created to train generalists. For sociologists, in particular, who have spent decades defining their domain (Weber, 1949; Millis, 1959) and who have finally distinguished themselves from social workers and other applied practitioners, their amalagamation with the generalists must be a source of ambivalence and irony.

Conclusion: Predictions for the Future

The outcomes described above are prevocative. If one were to predict the possibilities for eventual implementation of substantial sociological training in family medicine programs, one might best make the prediction from a sociological perspective. Specifically, it must be realized that the present day dilemma of family practice as a specialty is that on the one hand, it wants to be applied (in producing primary care physicians), while on the other, it has to establish an academic presence comparable to other specialties. Because the social science perspective in its curriculum offers family practice an academic identity (the goal of training being the treatment of illness in the context of family and community), it is perhaps the motivation for status and identity more than any clinical factors that eventually may bring about the integration of sociology into the family medicine curriculum.

In the next decade behavioral scientists will strengthen their foothold in the family medicine curriculum and become an integral part of the academic definition of family medicine. This process is enhanced by liberal federal funding and resources from foundations and other government agencies. However, it should not be expected that sociology or any other particular discipline within this emerging movement, whose strength lies in its collective identity, can afford to seek individual prominence and recognition.[3]

REFERENCES

Ad Hoc Committee on Education for Family Practice of the Council on Medical Education. Meeting the challenge of family practice. Chicago: American Medical Association, 1966.

Citizen's Commission on Graduate Medical Education. The graduate education of physicians. Chicago: American Medical Association, 1966.

The core content of family medicine. *GP*, 1966, *34*, 225-246.

Dubos, R. *Mirage of health*. Anchor Books, 1959.

Fleming, W. Teaching of family physicians by a department of preventive medicine. *Journal of the American Medical Association*, 1956, *161*, 711-713.

Haggard, H. W. *Devils, drugs and doctors*. New York: Harper and Bros., 1929.

Haynes, M. A. An approach to the teaching of family care. *Journal of the American Medical Association*, 1960, *173*, 1340-1341.

Holzner, B., & Marx, J. H. The transformation of a professional epistemic community: The emergence of family medicine and family health care. In B. Holzner, & J. H. Marx, *Knowledge application: The knowledge system in society*. Boston: Allyn and Bacon, 1979, 155-168.

Mills, C. W. *The Sociological Imagination*. New York: Oxford University Press, 1959.

National Commission on Community Health Services. *Health is a community affair*. Cambridge, MA: Harvard University Press, 1966.

Oates, R. P., & Feldman, H. A. Patterns of change in medical student career choices. *Journal of Medical Education*, 1974, *49*, 562-569.

Rardin, T. E. A reappraisal of today's family physician. *Journal of the American Medical Association*, 1962, *182*, 545-547.

Rardin, T. E. Family practice, an emerging specialty with an exciting future. *New Physician*, 1963, 153-163.

---

[3]For a provocative assessment of the possible demystifying impact of the emergence of the family medicine orientation (specifically the focus on the patient as a participating partner in the relationship with the family physician), see B. Holzner and J. H. Marx, "The Transformation of a Professional Epistemic Community: The Emergence of Family Medicine and Family Health Care", pp. 155-168 in B. Holzner and J. H. Marx, *Knowledge Application: The Knowledge System in Society*, Boston: Allyn and Bacon, 1979.

Shyrock, R. H. *The development of modern medicine*. Philadelphia: University of Pennsylvania Press, 1936.

Shyrock, R. H. *Medicine and society in America, 1660-1960*. New York: University Press, 1960.

Sigerist, H. *On the history of medicine*. New York: MD Publications, 1960.

Silver, G. *Family medical care*. Cambridge, MA: Harvard University Press, 1963.

Silver, G. Family practice: Resuscitation or reform? *Journal of the American Medical Association*, 1965, *183* (part 3), 188-189.

United States Department of Health, Education and Welfare. Public Health Service. National Institute of Health. National Institute of Child Health and Human Development. Behavioral sciences in medical education: A report of four conferences. D.H.E.W. Publication No. (NIH) 72-41, 1972.

Walsh, J. S. New specialty–Family practice. *Journal of the American Medical Association*, 1970, *212*, 1192-1193.

Weber, M. *The methodology of the social sciences*. Translated and edited by Edward A. Shils and Henry A. Finch (Trans. and Eds.). Glencoe, IL: The Free Press, 1949.

THE RELATIONAL MODEL IN FAMILY PRACTICE

Lynn P. Carmichael, MD
Joan S. Carmichael, PhD

Medical practitioners are interested in the care of patients and the treatment of their illnesses. In medical practice a favorable result is more important than how it is attained. However, an understanding of the process of medical care has valuable implications for health care delivery as well as the education of physicians.

One approach to understanding what goes on in medical practice is to develop a conceptual model. This has been done by Lazare (1973) to explain clinical psychiatry and by Friedson (1975) to study prepaid group practice. Based on systems theory, Engel (1980) developed the biopsychosocial model to take into account the missing dimensions of the dominant biomedical model. When using models it is important to keep in mind that they are intellectual interpretations and not factual descriptions of phenomena. Friedson (1975) alludes to this when he states, "But since they are solely models–which is to say logical constructs, aids to systematic thinking rather than descriptions–they are not embodied in pure form in any social policy or, for that matter in any productive enterprise." Lazare (1973) cautions: "(1) No model offers a complete explanation to the phenomena to which it addresses itself. (2) Any two conceptual models may offer alternative explanations for the same behavioral events. (3) In applying more than one conceptual model in treating a given patient, we must recognize the possibility of apparent contradictions."

In an attempt to gain a clearer understanding of family practice, three conceptual constructs are formulated: the clinical model, the relational model, and the adversarial model. This paper will be concerned principally with the relational model and will use the others to complete the picture of family practice.

Dr. L. Carmichael is family physician, and Professor and Chairperson, Department of Family Medicine, University of Miami School of Medicine, Miami, FL 33101.

Dr. J. Carmichael is Assistant Professor, Department of Epidemiology and Public Health, University of Miami School of Medicine.

Marriage & Family Review, Vol. 4(1/2), Spring/Summer 1981

The Content of General Medical Practice

Recent studies, most notably the National Ambulatory Medical Care Survey (De Lozier, 1975), provide insight into what has been called the content of family practice. An interpretation of this study is illustrated in Figure 1. As shown, in half of the ambulatory encounters with the family general practitioner, the patient has an illness for which there is objective evidence of physical pathology. In 15 of the 50 encounters the problem identified may result in significant impairment or death if left untreated. The adequate management of the disease in five of these patients (one-third of the progressive disorders) requires the involvement of other specialists and often hospitalization. In 10 of the 15 (two-thirds of progressive group), successful management is within the capability of the generalist (family practitioner). The approach to these progressive problems which result in a cure or control (either now or at some future time) by a pill or a procedure has been characterized as the clinical model.

The remaining 35 of the 50 encounters involving physical disease are for conditions that are self-limited, i.e., disorders to which the individual has successfully adapted. Self-limited diseases or injuries do not require medical intervention for complete resolution and are not associated with permanent disability or death. The role of physicians in self-limited problems is to provide relief of symptoms (e.g., prescribing codeine) and in some cases to hasten recovery (e.g., lancing a boil), but neither narcotics or surgery alter the final outcome, i.e., resolution without significant impairment.

Of the remaining 50 encounters in which there is no objective evidence of a biological base for the disturbance, 35 have behavioral manifestations of a disorder involving the emotions or feelings of the individual and are in the affective domain. These are referred to as psychosocial problems (P.S. in Figure 1). Prevention-oriented services such as checkups, prenatal care, and immunizations account for another 10 of the 50 encounters. Garfield (1970) has combined the psychosocial and the prevention groups into the "worried well." This term reflects the view that only the physically sick require medical attention. Cassel (1976) has dealt with those patients more kindly by pointing out that it is possible to have illness without disease. The remaining 5% of the visits seek medical services not for help but for administrative purposes (e.g., certification of disability). For this group the physician is placed in an adversary relationship to the patient, and most physicians find this role uncomfortable and troublesome.

FIGURE 1

CONTENT OF GENERAL MEDICAL PRACTICE

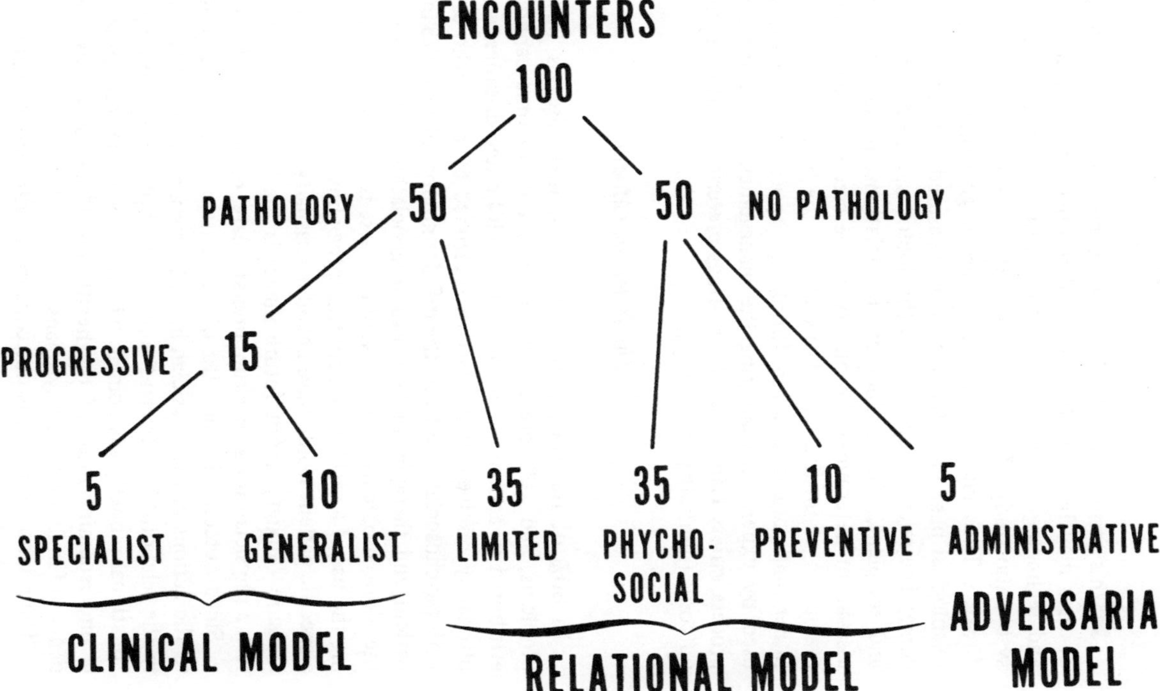

The Clinical Model

In this formulation the "clinical model" is restricted to patients whose diseases may be controlled or cured through advances in biomedical science and technology either at present or in the future. Biomedical science is the systematic study of the physical world in order to prevent, cure, or control diseases. Thus management of disease is goal oriented and springs from a teleological base in which success is measured in terms of the result or outcome. The relationship between the doctor and the patient is that of provider and recipient. The product of this relationship can be assessed, and this assessment determines the quality of the care provided. Parenthetically, the evaluation of medical care is usually on the basis of physician performance rather than patient response. Brook and Appel (1973) report that the criteria used by experts in evaluating the management of hypertension are of the process variety (laboratory tests, drugs prescribed) rather than dependent on outcome (morbidity, mortality).

The Relational Model

In 80% of the encounters (35% self-limited diseases, 35% psychosocial problems, and 10% preventive services) the outcome cannot be definitely attributed to actions of the physician. Self-limited disorders are by definition ultimately resolved. While success is claimed by those who care for patients with psychosocial problems, the infinite number of variables in the life of the patient and therapist make a causal association difficult to determine and, therefore, problematic. In prevention there is a statistical basis for championing the use of a vaccine or a contraceptive; however, there is no certainty that a specific patient would have become a casualty were it not for the preventive measure. Anxiety about future illness is the base of a patient's decision to seek a physician for a checkup, prenatal care, or other methods of prevention.

Since outcome in the 80% of encounters cannot be definitely attributed to the actions of the physician in caring for a specific patient, attention shifts to the relationship between the patient and physician. Consequently the term "relational model" was coined, which refers to the conceptual approach used in understanding most of the health and illness problems presented by patients to family practice physicians.

The relational model is not concerned with cure or control of disease but rather with the attention, support, and comfort the patient receives. The physician acts on the basis of what ought to be done. What ought to be done involves the rights of the patient and the duties of the physician. The relational model is concerned with the rightness or wrongness of the process or the action itself and not with the consequences of the therapeutic action. This model assumes action for social and affectual and not instrumental purposes. Concern is with feelings, relationships, and the skills to cope with mental and physical stress. The doctor and the patient become participants in this action and process criteria such as style, manner, and responsiveness are used for evaluation. The amount and type of care open to the relational model is determined by nondisease factors.

The Adversarial Model

The remaining 5% of the encounters involve patients seeking the services of a medical practitioner not because they want care for an illness but because they desire something only a physician is societally sanctioned to provide. Society, acting through legal and social mechanisms, has given the physician privileges to exercise control over certain medically related objects such as drugs, devices, and certificates. Examples are certification of disability for an injured worker or a narcotic prescription for a drug addict. The physician is placed in an adversary relationship to the patient and their relationship is often one of antagonists. The numbers may vary as laws and social mores change, but may be determined.

The various features of the three models are contrasted in Table 1. The remainder of this paper will explore various facets of the relational model and how it differs from the medical model.

Foundations

In general, there are two broad, opposing philosophies that guide much of our day-to-day activities. John Stuart Mill was one of the leading advocates of a teleological or utilitarian approach to action that has as its concern human values and goals. This philosophy maintains that what is right should result in the greatest good for the greatest number, and an act is not wrong or right in itself but is determined by the consequences of that act. The acts of a physician are good if they serve a societally determined goal such as relief of pain and cure or controlled disease. According to this philosophy the physician should make all necessary efforts to prolong life even in the face of a fatal illness, and may or may not inform the patient that the illness is fatal. Scientific medicine is goal directed and teleologically oriented.

Immanuel Kant championed a deontological system based on the assumption that persons have certain rights which should be respected. Persons are free agents and ought to act according to moral law. Kant's categorical imperative declares that a free moral agent must: (1) act as though the action

TABLE 1

COMPARISON OF CONCEPTUAL MODELS IN FAMILY PRACTICE

	CLINICAL MODEL	RELATIONAL MODEL	ADVERSARY MODEL
PERCENT ENCOUNTERS	15%	80%	5%
ORIENTATION	VALUES & GOALS	RIGHTS & DUTIES	PRIVILEGES & SANCTIONS
OBJECTIVE	CURE/CONTROL	CARE/COMFORT	CERTIFY
RELATIONSHIP	PROVIDER/RECIPIENT	PARTICIPANTS	ANTAGONISTS
EVALUATION	OUTCOME	PROCESS	STRUCTURE

were a universal law, (2) treat persons as ends and never as a "means merely" to other ends, and (3) consider every human being as one considers oneself. According to this philosophy open communication is the norm. For example, the patient has a right to know if one has a fatal illness and the physician has a moral obligation to inform the patient. When treating a patient, the patient as a free moral agent must consent to whatever therapy is given. Implied is the existence of a contract between doctor and patient. The philosophical foundation of the relational model is deontological.

There is also a behavioral disposition or ethological base to the relational model. This is the phenomena of maternal-infant bonding and social grooming so characteristic of primate societies. Newborns have a need to bond with mature functioning individuals if they are to survive in a hostile environment. Without another to feed, protect, and care for it, the newborn mammalian infant will die. The phenomenon of bonding has been well documented in animals and studies by Kennel and Klaus (1974) confirm its existence in humans. These studies demonstrate that maternal concern and infant weight gain are greater when time and circumstances allow considerable mother-infant interaction immediately after birth. The maternal-infant bond may be the prototype for all human relationships. This conditioning establishes the basis for forming future relationships and ultimately gives rise to the family. Circumstances that interfere with the establishment of the mother-infant bond in the immediate postnatal period may have significant effect on the infant's future ability to establish satisfying long-standing relationships.

One can speculate about the effect of modern obstetrical delivery techniques on present day society that is so marked by estrangement and violence. In 1947 Miller (1974) began a longitudinal study of infants and their families in Newcastle-On-Tyne. The infant mortality rate was 44 per 1000, and 50% of deliveries were in the home. Child abuse was not recognized or even acknowledged by Miller. Currently less than 2% of births are at home, infant mortality is 18 per 1000, and child abuse approaches the U.S. rate. It appears that hospital delivery reduces infant mortality but may also interfere with mother-infant bonding. Child abuse seems to be rare when bonding occurs. Fortunately this deficit in obstetrical practice is being corrected. Duff (1980) noted that birth is a family affair as the expression "in the family way" suggests, and increasingly, both parents are being involved in the delivery. Early physical and emotional contact with the newborn is being stressed, thus recognizing the critical nature of bonding for physical survival and social adjustment in later life.

The relational model has as part of its foundation the natural tendency of individuals to develop a bond. Evidence of this bond is seen in the phenomenon of social grooming in the primates. Grooming is more than simple skin care, although care of the skin by another animal is of considerable value to the one being groomed. Grooming is a social function that helps maintain social structure, relieves tension, and facilitates communication. The amount and form of grooming relates to social position, sex, age, stress, and condition. The relationship of grooming to health care has been well examined. Books by Morris (1967) and Tiger and Fox (1971) present fascinating and delightful insights into health and human behavior. While somewhat fanciful, it is interesting to speculate that most interaction between the doctor and the patient is but a highly stylized form of social grooming. This has led us to speak of "stroking and streaking in health care," the streakers being the 15% of patients that get all the attention from the medical model, and the strokers being the 80% who fill waiting rooms of family physicians. No doubt touching the patient relieves stress and the reduction in stress results in less disease. Perhaps the "laying on of hands" is not merely folklore or mysticism. Reinstituting the back rub as standard hospital procedure may balance the introduction of the computed axial tonography scanner. In the relational model, the good doctor is a good groomer.

Characteristics

To reflect on the physician or surgeon treating a patient with disease–the medical model–brings to mind such characteristics as authority, rationality, objectivity, and activity. Four elements of a different order characterize the relational model: affinity, intimacy, reciprocity, and continuity.

Affinity. A solo individual cannot bond; it takes two or more persons to form a bonding relationship. Bonds occur between persons, not between a person such as a physician and an abstraction such as disease or an object such as the microscope. The physician bonds with the patient, not with the disease. Affinity refers to the bond that links doctor and patient in the relational model.

Intimacy. Eating, sleeping, or having sex together does not in itself result in intimacy. Implied in intimacy is an openness and a willingness to acknowledge our vulnerability which leads to trust and acceptance. Intimacy is the trust a patient gives to the physician, and the physician's obligation is to use this for the patient's benefit. Intimacy is heightened by the opportunities for physical touching within the doctor-patient relationship.

Reciprocity. There is a reciprocal relationship between the doctor and patient that gives rise to an interdependency. This reliance on each other is not from weakness, but results in greater strength–just as the tepee is a stronger architectural structure than a single upright pole. Reciprocity is acknowledged by the physician when he says "my patient," and by the patient when he says "my doctor." The high collection rate by the family physician in private fee-for-service practice probably comes from reciprocity on the part of the patient. The patient pays the bill, not for service given, but rather for service that may be needed in the future.

Continuity. The patient and the physician recognize they have a past relationship and a reasonable expectation that it will continue. The patient does not have to formulate contingency plans for what to do if she/he becomes ill. Likewise, the physician accumulates information about the patient that may aid in the management of future problems. The development of continuity hinges on the duration, intensity, and quality of the relationship.

These four elements of the relational model–affinity, intimacy, reciprocity, and continuity–also characterize family relationships. Carmichael (1976) suggested the word "family" in family medicine refers to the type of relationship existing between patient and doctor rather than the family as a social unit.

Family doctors may care for all members of a family, but rarely if ever does the family as a unit become the patient or object of care. Indeed, good doctors care for the individual in the context of the family or with a family orientation. In those 80% of the encounters encompassed within the relational model, the doctor has a "family" type relationship with the patient. The family in family medicine refers to process (the doctor-patient relationship) rather than to entity (the family).

Competencies

Fried (1974) has written about rights in personal care. These rights may be translated into competencies the physician needs in the relational model. These skills are of a different order from the medical model which stresses the perceptive, cognitive, and manipulative skills. The competencies in the relational model derive from the rights of patients and duties of physicians. These are the elements of personal care listed by Fried, and we draw heavily on his description.

Lucidity. The physician has a duty to inform the patient of the relevant details about his/her problem. Lucidity is a constructive good, and to deny the patient full information is to treat the patient not as a person, but merely as a means. Fried states, "Denial of lucidity is a sufficient condition for a relation of dominance, and that in itself is a violation of rights" (1974, p. 101).

Autonomy. The patient and physician are both autonomous, free agents and neither can abuse the liberty of the other. Neither the patient nor the physician should be treated or treat against his/her will. Autonomy is not simply *allowing* but *insisting* that the participants in the relationship decide for themselves after full and understandable explanation.

Fidelity. The physician and patient engender expectations in each other. These expectations need to be respected, and coercion and intimidation on both parts must be avoided. As Fried says, "Deliberately to disappoint such expectations is a form of deceit" (1974, p. 102).

Humanity. Physicians frequently deal with patients whose physiology or psychology is disturbed. The use of the previously mentioned three competencies in a patient with a high fever, acute agitation, or moribund state may not be understood by the patient. In such instances the physician looks to family members and others for protection of the patient's rights until the patient is once again in full control of his/her sensibilities. The use of humanity in dealing with patients is the vaguest of all four competencies. There are few guidelines and many critics.

Summary

These three models were developed from a retrospective analysis of encounters in family practice and should not be taken as operational methods for providing care or managing patients' problems. They are, instead, a conceptual approach to understanding what goes on in general medical practice. However, there are practical applications for the planning, implementation, and evaluation of health care programs and for the education of health professionals that have important humanistic and economic considerations.

Advances in the biomedical sciences have lead to the cure and control of many diseases that often in the past caused significant disability or death. This success leads us to suspect pathology where it does not exist, to undertake dangerous investigation and intervention in disorders in which the outcome is rarely in doubt, and to convert problems of living into medical diseases. The inappropriate application of the techniques useful in the clinical model to problems belonging to the relational model results in excessive testing, prescribing, hospitalization, and operative procedures. The goal orientation of curative medicine places a higher premium on the ends or outcome of treatment than the means or process of care. This carries with it the continued denial of patients' rights to autonomy, lucidity, fidelity, and humanity. Comprehension is needed on the part of all sectors of the health field as well as the public that the diagnostic and therapeutic methods associated with the clinical model constitute only a small part of the work of the family doctor. Continued failure to do so is already having dire consequences through the abasement of human dignity and the escalation of health care costs.

REFERENCES

Brook, R., & Appel, F. Quality and care assessment: Choosing a method for peer review. *New England Journal of Medicine*, 1973, *288*, 1323-1329.

Carmichael, L. P. The family in medicine: Process or entity? *Journal of Family Practice*, 1973, *3*(5), 562-563.

Cassell, E. Illness and disease. *Hastings Center Report VI*. 1976, 27-37.

De Lozier, J. *National ambulatory medical care survey 1973*. Summary DHEW Publication No. 1772 Series 13, Number 76. 1975, Washington, DC: National Center for Health Statistics.

Duff, R. Care in childbirth and beyond. *New England Journal of Medicine*, 1980, *302*, 685-686.

Engel, G. The clinical application of the biopsychosocial model. *The American Journal of Psychiatry*, 1980, *137*(5), 535-544.

Fried, C. *Medical experimentation: Personal integrity and social policy*. New York: American Elsevier, 1974.

Friedson, E. *Doctoring together*. New York: American Elsevier, 1975.

Garfield, S. The delivery of medical care. *Scientific American*, 1970, 15-23.

Kennel, J., & Klaus, M. Maternal behavior after early and extended postpartum contact. *Developmental Medicine and Child Neurology*, 1974, *16*, 172-179.

Lazare, A. Hidden conceptual models in clinical psychiatry. *New England Journal of Medicine*, 1973, *288*, 345-350.

Miller, F. *The school years in Newcastle-Upon-Tyne*. London: Oxford University Press, 1974.

Morris, D. *The naked ape*. New York: Dell, 1967.

Tiger, L., & Fox, R. *The imperial animal*. New York: Dell, 1971.

THE CONSUMER AND FAMILY PHYSICIAN RELATIONSHIP: POWER, AUTONOMY, COMPLIANCE, AND NEGOTIATION

Morton M. Warner, PhD

Introduction

Research on the development and activities of professional groups has become increasingly popular. Studies in the past, [for example, those by Carr-Saunders and Wilson (1933), Parsons (1949), Merton (1957), and Goode (1957)] have, however, tended to relegate the role of the patient or client to a position of minor importance. It is perhaps since the period of the mid-1960s that a wave of consumerism is found in almost every sphere of life.

Background to the Study

The data which form the basis of this discussion comes from a study initiated by the Lay Advisory and Research Committees of the British Columbia Chapter of the College of Family Physicians of Canada. It recognizes that the practice of family medicine cannot exist without clients and that those clients will often have markedly different ideas about what they want and expect from those ideas supposedly held by the professionals they consult. The origins and development of a consumer group in the medical field are of more than passing interest because they represent, in this instance, a first attempt to plan consumer input into the education process of both intending and practicing family physicians or general practitioners.* In March 1970, the

---

Dr. Warner is Associate Professor and Director, Graduate Program in Health Services Planning, Department of Health Care and Epidemiology, University of British Columbia, 2075 Wesbrook Mall, Vancouver, B.C. V6Y 1W5, Canada.

This research was completed under funding by Health & Welfare Canada, Grant No. 610-21-18. Acknowledgement is given to the assistance of Ms. Gay Christophedes and Dr. Tim Cramer of the Univeristy of British Columbia, to the College of Family Physicians of Canada, and to the Lay Advisory Committee to the British Columbia Chapter.

---

*See Appendix "On General Practice and Family Medicine."

Board of Directors of the College of Family Physicians of Canada passed a resolution to explore the possible value of the attachment of a group of consumers. In June of the same year, the Board of Directors of the British Columbia Chapter passed its own resolution that "the British Columbia Chapter explore the establishment of a Lay Advisory Committee to study priorities from the consumer point of view." In the late summer of 1970, a Lay Advisory Committee (LAC) was established under the auspices of the British Columbia Chapter, its terms of reference being two-fold: (1) to consider the medical needs** of the consumer, and (2) the availability of medical services as they relate to the College's position concerning education and manpower.

The British Columbia Lay Advisory Committee developed on an ad hoc basis initially through consultation with local voluntary organizations, but more frequently through members joining the Committee having heard about it through friends. The result was a high turnover during the first year. The group was chaired by a school counselor and initially included an old age pensioner, two students, housewives, church people, men and women from different professional groups, and two people who were at that time receiving Social Assistance.

Rather than acting in formal committee fashion, the group spent the early months learning about various aspects of health care and discovering that both they and other members of the public to whom they spoke were either totally uninformed or often misinformed about matters pertaining to health. The group used this period in an educative way and invited persons from various health disciplines to meet with them in order to obtain, first hand, a view of the attitudes that health professionals held toward each other and toward health care, and particularly to get a better understanding of the stance that was adopted towards family medicine. The British Columbia Chapter, for purposes of liaison, always had one of their members in attendance. It is important to note that this physician took a totally nondirective approach and allowed the group to set its own pattern of behavior, to come to its own understanding of the problems, and only gave responses when direction or information was requested.

The single most important shift that occurred during the first 6 months was the capacity of the members of the LAC to move from the particular to the general. At first they related their own experiences, but later moved to developing a patchwork of issues that were of concern and that could be generalized as representing problems vis-a-vis medicine in particular and

---

**"Medical needs" was later translated by the LAC to mean "health needs in the area of Family Medicine."

health care in total. A further understanding was gained that people from different backgrounds were likely to be looking for different things from their family physician, and that if a sufficiently varied and representative body of opinion was to be gathered, than an approach must be adopted other than the meeting of an ad hoc committee. The overall task of reporting within the broad terms of reference of the National Chapter was soon recognized as impossible, since no adequate formula existed as to the representativeness of the committee. Consequently, the survey research method was adopted and appropriate instruments developed through liaison with a local university. The emphasis, however, remained upon producing questions that substantively represented consumer concerns, not concerns that professionals believe consumers to have.

The Development of Hypotheses

An important theme of the College of Family Physicians is education of its membership; thus, the major hypothesis centers around education and the relationship between family physicians and their patient-clients that presently exists, and that might exist in the future. The wording is as follows:

> That because the norms of operation of the family physician are likely to be in conflict with the expectations and needs as perceived by his present and future clientele, the family physician will not achieve his maximum usefulness until more is known about relevant training for his current task and/or appropriate reeducation of the public occurs.

From this, a model can be suggested. It is not one in which client and practitioner are separate entities, but rather a system in which representatives of the medical profession practice in local communities of prospective clients (Parsons, 1954). Practitioners claim that their skills are so esoteric that the patient is in no position to evaluate them; this is described as the prerogative of their peers. But the practitioner will be evaluated by the patient, albeit on an unprofessional basis with nonprofessional criteria. Hence, practice may consist of an interaction between two different and sometimes conflicting sets of norms (Freidson, 1966).

Congruency between the responses of family physicians and consumers in a number of areas–autonomy, compliance, power, and negotiation–is the central theme of this discussion. It was postulated that incongruencies would exist and be of sufficient dimension to throw into question some basic assumptions about the characteristic of total dependency of the patient role.

The Development of the Data Collection Instruments

Conceptualization

During the period when the LAC was beginning to form, the author, a medical sociologist, was, through invitation by the group, involved on a participant-observation basis. The process of the meetings was observed, information was fed back, and additional assistance was given that helped in comprehending the matters to be studied.

As a result, a number of areas–utilization, access and the organization of family practice, general availability, appointment systems, type of office, house calls, availability of laboratory systems, and atmosphere–all items which, in Donabedian's terms (1968), might be referred to as "issues of structure," emerged.

A second area of interest focused around the total or generic needs that patients who approach family physicians often have. The job specification described by The Royal College of General Practitioners (1969) comes closest in detailing the way that the committee felt a family physician might function:

> The general practitioner is a doctor who provides personal, primary and continuing medical care to individuals and families....He accepts the responsibility for making an initial decision on every problem his patient may present to him....His diagnosis will be composed in physical, psychological and social terms. He will intervene educationally, preventively and therapeutically to promote his patient's health (p. 358).

It is clear that a family physician who has to deal adequately with the total needs of patients must have at hand a wide range of skills other than those of strictly medical origin. Only then would the connections between an individual's behavior in health and disease, and his relationships with other significant individuals who form his social environment become evident. In essence, the group agreed with the Australian Medical Association's statement (1970): "For the doctor who is able to use sociological and psychological frames of reference, much work which previously seemed unintelligible or trivial and often irremedial and frustrating can become intelligible, more manageable and more rewarding" (p. 41).

Another area considered to be of importance is the role of the family physician in dealing with nonmedical problems and, where these problems are of a multidimensional nature, his ability to work with others involved in the delivery of care. These potential demands have been considered by various groups of general practitioners and their conclusions are clear: "The days of the do-it-all-himself doctor are over and in general practice as elsewhere the work to be done is best managed by a team or group of doctors and their nursing and other colleagues working together, each adding their skills and expertise to the best way of helping the patient." (Royal College of General Practitioners, 1973, p. 42).

The Australian Medical Association (1970) also takes a specific stance:

> Some patients, particularly those with chronic and multiple disabilities, need more than individual episodes of care. They require planned programs of management, which will involve teams of varying composition for prolonged periods, and their relationships within the team will vary at different phases of such a program (p. 41).

The list of concerns so far is lengthy, but its consideration is important as a precursor to the central theme of the discussion—the relationship that exists between family physicians and their patients in all its facets. Essentially, the concern was directed at the consumer's dilemma of wanting, at one and the same time, control over his own life, despite the decrease of rights and obligations customary during a period of sickness and the concomitant increase in dependence on the family physician. The sense of powerlessness associated with this process was at the core of the discussions. An editorial in *The Journal of the Royal College of General Practitioners* (1974) puts the case very clearly when it describes the vulnerability of patients as they approach the medical care system:

> Such vulnerability creates a responsibility for doctors—both individually and collectively....Sometimes in the past, doctors have adopted unthinkingly a rigid and authoritarian position. The challenge for general practice is now to evolve—and evolve quickly—a relationship which secures for the patient appropriate power and responsibility whilst retaining for the profession, power to innovate and to improve quality....The management of a patient—especially in general practice—is not now a short simple technical procedure, but an exercise in options.... Many of the choices cannot be decided by the doctor alone, but each needs to be proposed and discussed with the patient and often with the family. All this means that the doctor becomes less authoritarian and less rigid....Patients in the future will be required to participate more and so accept much more responsibility (p. 1).

Questionnaire Development

Two questionnaires–one for consumers, the other for family physicians–were developed consecutively. The main feature of this process was that the physician questionnaire was a mirror image of that developed for the consumer group rather than vice versa. Four drafts of the consumer questionnaire were produced by the medical sociologist, and these were constantly reviewed by the LAC to ascertain that the issues stated were indeed the issues previously discussed, and that the wording employed would be palatable and understandable to a wide range of consumers in the community. Following this activity, the physician questionnaire was devised with special attention being given to comparability of wording to ensure similarity between the dimensions to be examined. Ideally, it would have been desirable to sample a selection of family physicians together with a selection of their own patients, but this was not possible due to the fact that the health care system itself allows freedom of choice on the part of patients and the possibility that a person may see a number of doctors in any given time span. It was, therefore, felt adequate to sample independently within the same city area.

Questionnaire Content and Educational Objectives

One important reason for the existence of the LAC is their consideration of the practice of family medicine and their subsequent recommendations for the training of family physicians. The method proposed to achieve this end was to develop a survey that would better an understanding of the perceptions that patients have of the "structural" and "process" issues as they relate to family medicine. It was only after the group had formulated their specific concerns that any attempt was made to relate these to the educational objectives laid down by the College of Family Physicians of Canada (1973).

Results

Demographic

It should be noted that in the case of consumers, "not eligible" represents the households where, after three call-backs, no respondent could be contacted who was 15-years-old or older, or where no method could be found to communicate either using a reliable translator from survey team or through close relatives. The interviewers were, in fact, given total freedom to interview whoever came to the door as long as he/she fell within the eligible all range.

TABLE 1. RESPONSE RATES OF CONSUMERS AND PHYSICIANS

CONSUMERS	
Completed	551 (68.3%)
Refused	233 (28.4%)
Not Eligible	28 (3.4%)
No English	9 (1.1%)
N=	821 (101.2%)

FAMILY PHYSICIANS	
Completed	86 (94.5%)
Out of Area	2 (2.2%)
Refused	3 (3/2%)
N=	91 (99.9%)

Error due to rounding

Graphs 1 and 2 illustrate the distributions by age and sex of the consumer and physician respondents. As expected, the consumers cover a wider age range and are predominantly female in comparison to the physicians.

Because much of what was asked of consumers relied on their memory of events, only those who had had contact in the 12 months prior to the survey personally or through their families were included. This represented 88.2% of the survey population. The median number of visits per year was about three, which for a fee-for-service system is interesting and comparable to results displayed from British studies under a capitation system. (Fry, 1972; Stein, 1967).

There is an interesting, but expected, differentiation in the utilization by socioeconomic status delineated by the Blishen Scale (Blishen, 1967), as seen in Table 2. People in the upper socioeconomic groups tend to use their family physician less (it may be that they use specialists more), and at the high utilization level (nine+visits per year), the lower socioeconomic groups tend to predominate.

The Dynamics of the Doctor-Consumer-Patient Relationship

Any piece of research that sets out, at least in part, to examine the doctor-patient rather than the doctor-consumer relationship is faced with a dilemma. In fact, in the area of family medicine, it is rarely possible to carry out wide-scale surveys on people who are actually undergoing treatment. Rather, it is more likely that the interviewed group will be consumers of family medicine. That is to say, in the relatively distant past they will have had some experience of seeking family physician care, but that at the time of being interviewed they will not actually be sick. This distinction is important, especially when trying to make an assessment of the attitudes, feelings, and dimensions that are involved in the consumer-patient-physician relationship. When a person is well, he has general control over his own life and is not forced into a dependency role upon a physician. He more or less has the option as to how he wishes to relate to his environment or to his family, and in what fashion he will carry out his work. However, sickness and the patient role bring with them a change in rights and obligations. Society has deemed

GRAPH 1. AGE DISTRIBUTION OF CONSUMERS AND PHYSICIANS, BY PERCENT

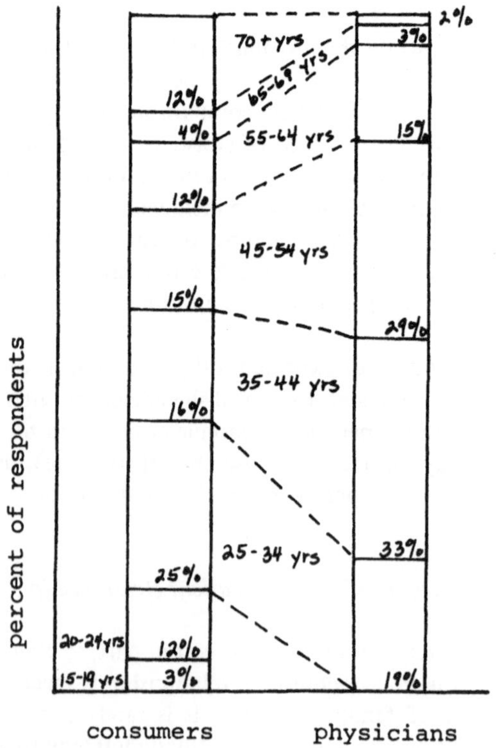

GRAPH 2. SEX DISTRIBUTION OF CONSUMERS AND PHYSICIANS, BY PERCENT

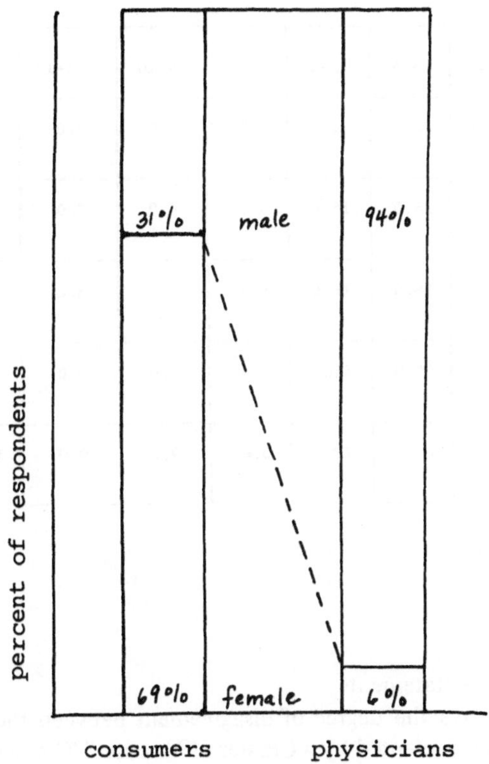

that persons who are sick and who are certified as such by a physician, do not have to work, at least for a period of time; they are expected to transfer their energies toward getting well. For episodes of time, then, governments are prepared to support a person financially, employers are willing to give sick leave, and relatives will look after the patient.

A series of attitudinal statements pertaining to various aspects of the relationship were put to the consumer and physician groups. The responses indicate the degree of congruence or incongruence; from this potential areas of conflict can be identified and can be dealt with at the educational and practice levels.

Table 3 was developed by making a comparison of the responses of physicians and consumers.

TABLE 2. NUMBER OF CONTACTS WITH FAMILY DOCTOR IN PREVIOUS 12 MONTHS BY SOCIOECONOMIC GROUPING -- BY PERCENT

	None	1-2	3-4	5-6	7-8	9-10	11-12	13+	% N
I	8.0	35.0	22.0	11.0	4.0	5.0	5.0	12.0	100 (199)
II	5.0	37.0	26.0	15.0	3.0	4.0	3.0	7.0	100 (121)
III	6.0	44.0	19.0	14.0	6.0	1.0	3.0	8.0	100 (73)
IV	9.0	51.0	19.0	6.0	3.0	3.0	0.0	10.0	100 (70)
un-known	9.0	35.0	17.0	13.0	0.0	9.0	0.0	17.0	100 (23)

I = Low SES

IV = High SES

Column I lists the statements.

Column II displays the degree of disagreement between the responses of both groups and is represented by a Cramer's "V-score." The higher the score, the greater the level of disagreement.

Column III ranks the Cramer's V-score from highest to lowest of disagreement.

Column IV concentrates upon the direction of agreement towards the statement, indicating whether consumers (←) or physicians (→) agree most with the statement made of whether each individual aspect of the relationship is patient-initiated (P.I.) or doctor-initiated (D.I.), as shown in Column V.

Column VI compares the responses of Columns IV and V. One star indicates that the direction of agreement was from the physicians (→), yet from Column V it can be seen that it was a patient-initiated aspect (P.I.). Two stars show that the direction of agreement came from the consumers (←), and yet in Column V the issue was seen to be doctor-initiated (D.I.).

Column VII gives an arbitrary but rational title to each attitudinal aspect that was considered where potential conflicts had been isolated, and final results show that issues relating to autonomy were ranked 1, 2, 4, 6, and 9, conflicts over office organization 11 and 14, and conflicts over the character of the physician 3 and 5.

Discussion

Autonomy

The fact that problems exist around this area indicates the confused nature of the role of the consumer/patient. In family medicine, probably as in no other form of doctoring, there exists a very high proportion of people with minor ailments who have the opportunity to act quite independently. Non-compliance to the suggestions of their physicians and an essential wish to remain autonomous are two important patient characteristics. Family physicians, who are presently trained in an excessively specialist-oriented world, with much of their experience being gained in hospitals where patients are in a far more dependent position, will need to understand to a greater extent the feelings of autonomy that patients in the ambulatory care area exhibit.

But doctors, too, are an autonomous group. Some of the following quotations given verbally at the time of the questionnaires' administration help display this.

Item: Patients who will not follow the doctor's advice.
Response: "If they don't follow advice, I tell them to see another doctor."
Item: To ensure continuity of care, a patient should be seen even though the doctor may be short of time.
Response: "Yes, but he should be seen at the doctor's convenience."
Item: The doctor's manner is not important as long as he is careful.
Response: "He won't have many patients, but it won't affect his treatment."
Item: It is not important that the doctor should like the patient.
Response: "If I don't like them, I tell them. I don't want to treat them if I don't like them."
Item: Patients generally like to be told exactly what to do, not given alternative courses of action.

TABLE 3. COMPARISON OF RESPONSE PHYSICIANS AND CONSUMERS ON ASPECTS OF DOCTOR-PATIENT RELATIONSHIP

I. Attitudinal Statement	II. Cramer's V	III. Rank order of Cramer's V	IV. Direction of Agreement: Consumer ← Physician → Similar ↑	V. Patient-initiated/ Doctor-initiated	VI. Conflict	VII. Area of Conflict
More important to respect than like	.25256	7	↑	PI		
Family Physician should give prescription patient wants	.31754	4	→	PI	*	Autonomy
Doctor should be firm rather than coddle	.39743	1	←	DI	**	Autonomy
Being a doctor should not be only reason for respect	.35813	3	→	PI	*	Character of Physician
Expect to see my doctor, not another, even though he is short of time	.18890	11	→	PI	*	Office Organization
Manner not as important as skill	.3635	5	←	DI	**	Character of Physician
Phone advice should be avoided	.06136	19	↑	DI		
If problem is serious expect to be referred, even if my Family Doctor is competent	.37375	2	←	DI	**	Autonomy
Family doctor should use discretion in telling patients of serious illness	.25763	6	←	DI	**	Autonomy

TABLE 3. CONTINUED

Patients should be told what to do, not given alternatives	.21189	8	←	PI		
Family Doctor would give me a choice of specialists	.14006	13	↑	PI		
Family Doctor should be like a friend	.12426	15	↑	DI		
Would like Family Doctor's help in explaining serious illness to family	.09294	18	↑	DI		
Answering services should be used as little as possible	.13074	14	←	DI	**	Office Organi-zation
Patients should be left to follow advice, not supervised	.19116	10	←	PI		
Most important treatment often sympathy	.14157	12	→	DI		
Business-like offices inspire confidence	.12146	16	→	DI		
Wrong to let patients think Family Physician can do all things	.20244	9	←	DI	*	Autonomy
Important for Family Physician to show he cares	.10472	17	↑	DI		

Response: "You don't give the patient a choice. The person who wrote this question does not understand what being a doctor is all about. You tell a patient what to do."
Item: When should a family doctor give a full explanation of the patient's problems to the patient?
Response: "I never tell everything to a patient, only what they should know."

While these quotations do not represent the attitude taken by family physicians as a whole, they are somewhat characteristic of the attitudes that are generated in some of the more specialized areas of medical care where compliance equals dependence. This may be the situation, too, for some patients in the general practice setting, but it should be recognized that at different times compliance may equal something other than dependence. Deutsch (1971) makes some useful suggestions that may help, in part, to alleviate this problem:

> The patient who must bare himself physically and psychologically in front of his physician will see him as an omnipotent parental figure. This transference of feelings is often accompanied by some regression and infantilization. The physician should be aware that his attitudes may color and strengthen aspects of the transference and should discourage excessive infantilization in patients. Consultations with other physicians will modify the patient's perceptions of the doctor's omnipotence and thus will reduce the hostility at any failure in treatment. When doctors make referrals to specialists, they should explain the basis of their choice. Ultimately, doctors must try to achieve the perfect balance between closeness and distance, between human concern and professional objectivity (p. 923-924).

Patient-Consumer Compliance

Communication in lay terms is critical if there is to be any high level of understanding on the part of the patient of what is required if he is to become well. Riley (1966) conducted a study to find out how certain instructions given to a patient by a doctor might be interpreted by the patient. Questions to the patients related to dietary instruction, an area where the understanding could be measured with relative ease. The results show that a large area of ambiguity existed for the patient where doctors felt that straightforward instructions had been given. Golden and Johnston (1970) completed a study in a similar vein: through the use of tape-recorded interviews, patients were questioned by a third party after doctors had given their explanations and left the room. Conditions that interfered with an adequate understanding of what the physician had said included the anxiety of the patient about what was being told to him, as well as his intelligence, prior experience with the problem at hand, and the number of opportunities given to question his medical informant. Factors affecting the physician's ability to communicate clearly related primarily to the clarity and simplicity of his language, his own anxiety about what he was telling the patient, and his seeming unwillingness to provide opportunities for patient feedback that might indicate patient comprehension. This last item is open to question: is feedback deliberately not sought because of the amount of time the physician has or because physicians in general feel that they communicate so well that misunderstanding is impossible?

Some conclusions are clear. If the physician-patient relationship is not developed sufficiently and if communication does not operate at the highest level, then the likely effectiveness of any treatment that is prescribed will be seriously negated; additionally, the level of satisfaction on the part of the patient regarding the interaction will also be jeopardized.

What Should Patients Be Told?

This is an area of such contention that it is difficult to find any writer who expresses unreservedly the opinion that all patients should be told everything about life-threatening illness. At the other end of the spectrum, Vaisrub (1971), for example, even suggests that it is detrimental for patients to be informed about their terminal illness. He goes on to say that it is not always sinful and harmful to withhold the information from the patient.

> Many patients may not be able to bear the burden of the known imminence of death, and the knowledge may kill them spiritually....To date no mortal has received a divine estimate of his remaining days on earth and nature has not provided any such information either. In making the revelation to his patient, then, the physician sets himself above nature and plays Super God (p. 588).

Kram and Coldwell (1969) suggest that the patient's denial of the seriousness of his illness is mainly for his own benefit, but others have suggested that a physician should be more actively engaged in the death process. Kubler-Ross (1970) states that patients can be helped to accept their death with peace, and that terminal patients often express the wish that they had been told earlier of their condition in order to save the tormenting anxiety of not knowing. Wahl (1969) goes so far as to suggest that patients should be allowed to plan for the future, for themselves, and for family members in order to have a sense of continuum through their survivors.

Some other results from the present study indicate that 50% of the family physicians would never give a full explanation to the patient and another 30% would only give it on the insistence of the patient. There is, then, clearly a discretionary element on the part of the physician about the problem or its seriousness. Just as doctors displayed a concern about their level of discretion, so too did the consumers, but to a somewhat greater extent. When the issue finally came down the line, 60% of the consumers wanted the physician to use his discretion, while 40% wanted more patient autonomy.

"If the patient insists, one would always explain."
"Telling a patient depends entirely on the patient."
"I never tell everything to a patient, only what he should know."
"No point telling a patient if it is serious and will upset them a great deal, even if the patient does insist."
"If they ask, I always tell them the truth."
"Don't tell patients about incurable diseases."

Negotiation

A major area of incongruence exists in the amount of autonomy a patient in the primary medical care situation can have, at the same time allowing a physician to have reasonable confidence that any treatment he recommends will be complied with. A greater understanding on the part of the family physicians about the capacity of each and every one of their patients to handle his own life, the individual's coping ability, and his need for autonomy will allow a process of negotiation over autonomy to occur in a positive fashion.

While the issue of autonomy, at the present time, seems to be one that should cause concern, there is the highest possibility that practicing family physicians and residents in family practice programs can learn to negotiate more skillfully with patients over the needs that the patient has rather than merely to relate to the physicial diseases that exist. Autonomy and compliance as they relate to serious illness will continue to be a problem, but here too individuals have different capacities, support mechanisms, and degrees of willingness to deal with the issues at hand. Again, a willingness on the part of the family physician to negotiate will increase the autonomy and power that many people feel is necessary in order to maintain a sense of utility and self-worth.

Organizational Issues

Consumers of health care in a time of increased geographical mobility and increased specialization among health professionals and health facilities no longer are likely to receive care that exhibits continuity or genericism. Gone is the time of which Emily Carr (1942) writes so intriguingly in early Canada:

> When Victoria was young, specialists had not been invented–the family doctor did you all over. You did not have a special doctor for each part. Doctor Helmcken attended to all our ailments–Father's gout, our stomachaches; he even told us what to do once when the cat had fits. If he was wanted in a hurry he got there in no time and did not wait for you to become sicker so that he could make a bigger cure....He was very thin, very active, very cheery....Dr. Helmcken knew each part of every one of us. He could have taken us to pieces and put us together again without mixing up any of our legs or noses or anything (p. 199-201).

In contrast to this, Barlow (1971, p. 925) states that in our age of super-specialization and high standards of patient care, the rapport that used to exist between doctor and patient has been lost. Doctors are so concerned with the physical state of a patient that they often overlook his mental state.

Wolfe and Badgley (1972) have suggested that "the duration of the doctor-patient relationship is determined in part by a population's mobility and by the movement of doctors" (p. 72). To this can be added the freedom of choice that is exercised by patients attending any physician and the organization of a practice itself, which may demand that a patient see different doctors at different times if a practice is to run smoothly. Over and above this, Stevens (1974, p. 6-7), when describing in detail the brief encounter between family physician and patient, further highlights the problem of continuity of care. It is expected, on one hand, that the practitioner will have a continuous understanding of the dynamics that are involved in the delicate interrelationships that exist, while on the other hand, amid these complexities remains the fact that relationships between family physicians and patients are often fleeting and of short duration. He concludes by suggesting that "there can be few encounters where so much active psychic and intellectual work is done as in a difficult consultation. It is a process requiring training, great discipline, and a rigorous approach."

But what of family medicine in the future? What challenges are emerging, both at the practice and educational levels, that might change its relationship with its clientele?

While it is difficult to foresee an end to the one-to-one treatment relationship, it is possible to forecast a de-emphasis in the light of health field concept proposals (Lalonde, 1974, p. 31). Through its medical care financing, the government of Canada is promoting preventive care modalities. Conceptually, if this is to be successful, *patients* will no longer abrogate responsibility for themselves and their diseases, nor will the task demand upon them continue to be reduced by physician activity. Rather, there will be a requirement of increased *person* performance while healthy, with a cooptation of physician or other health professional skills to maintain that state of health. In this self-help situation, power, autonomy, compliance, and negotiation take on a new light.

At the present time there is little evidence to suggest that medical schools in Canada are responding to this challenge. Family medicine, however, is in a good position to act by extending its holistic approach to include environmental, occupational, and life-style concerns. To do so will place it further at risk: patients do not understand the current emphasis upon total family care, and faculties of medicine tend to give prestige to departments that concentrate upon the instrumental concerns of the specialties.

The Zeitgeist is clear and relationships will change. Family medicine must lead and not merely respond to those changes.

Conclusions

The classic doctor-patient relationship viewed in terms of illness versus health, compliance versus control, or passivity versus activity is being tested in a new way as relationships become more transient, as consumers receive a level of education allowing for discriminatory or differential decision-making, where continuity of care is reduced due to specialized professional behavior, and because the spirit of the times demands an emphasis upon prevention rather than cure.

In the family medicine field in particular, many nonmedical problems are presented by patients which involve mutual participation rather than passivity and where the concepts of health and illness are changing and do not have preselective criteria from which a continuum can easily be developed. For example, in dealing with drug behavior among teenagers, the family physician may find himself in a dilemma of wanting the teenager to comply to a dependency relationship in the initial stages of treatment, but recognizing that the essential ingredient of compliance may, at some later point, be independence. Additionally, the criteria used for treatment may not be medically normative but more societally normative and subject to constant shifts and changes.

Feelings on the part of consumers of a need for autonomy, power, and a possibility of negotiation regarding many aspects of care in the family medicine situation are clear. The advantages for consumers and family physicians relate to increased communication possibilities and a greater compliance—the physician complying by providing treatment appropriate to his patients' needs and the patient complying to appropriate treatment—which comes from a mutually bargained approach.

REFERENCES

Australian Medical Association. General practice and its future in Australia. Report No. 1 of the Australian Medical Association Study Group on Medical Planning, 1970.

Barlow, M. R. The forgotten human being—The patient. *South African Medical Journal*, 1971, *45*, 925-926.

Blishen, B. R. A socio-economic index for occupations in Canada. *Canadian Review of Sociology and Anthropology*, 1967, 4-41.

Carr-Saunders, A. M., & Wilson, P. A. *The professions*. Oxford: Clarendon Press, 1933.

Carr, E. *The book of small*. Oxford University Press, 1942.

College of Family Physicians of Canada. Canadian family medicine: Educational objectives for certification in family medicine. 1973.

Deutsch, L. The difficult patient in medical practice. *Journal of the Medical Society of New Jersey*, 1971, *68*, 923-924.

Donabedian, A. Promoting quality through evaluating the process of patient care. *Medical Care*, 5, 1968, *3*, 181-202.

Freidson, E. Client control and medical practice. In Scott, W. R. & Volkhart, E. H. (Eds.), *Medical care: Readings in the sociology of medical institutions*. 1966, 259-271.

Fry, J. Twenty-one years of general practice—Changing patterns. *Journal of the Royal College of General Practitioners*, 1972, *22*, 521-528.

Golden, J. L., & Johnston, G. D. Problems of distortion. In Doctor-patient communications, *Psychiatry and Medicine*, 1970, *1*, 127-149.

Goode, W. J. Community within a community: The professions. *American Sociological Review*, 1957, 194-200.

Knox, J. P. E. The new general practice - II. British Medical Association, 1970.

Kram, C., & Coldwell, J. M. The dying patient. *Psychosomatics*, 1969, *10*, 293-295.

Kubler-Ross, E. The care of the dying—Whose job is it? *Psychiatry and Medicine*, 1970, *1*, 103-107.

Lalonde, M. A new perspective on the health of Canadians: A working document. Government of Canada, 1974.

Merton, R. K. Some preliminaries to a sociology of medical education. In Merton, R. K., Reader, G., & Kendall, P. L. (Eds.), *The student physician*. Harvard University Press, 1957, 3-79.

Parsons, T. The professions and social structure. In *Essays in social theory pure and applied.* Glencoe: The Free Press, 1949, 185-189.
Parsons, T. The social system. Glencoe: The Free Press. 1954, 428-473.
Riley, C. S. Patient understanding of doctor's instructions. *Medical Care*, 1966, *4*, 34-37.
Royal College of General Practitioners. The educational needs of the future general practitioner. Reports from *General Practice*, 1969, 18.
Royal College of General Practitioners. Present state and future needs of general practice. Reports from *General Practice*, 1973, *3*, 16.
Royal College of General. Practitioners Patient Power, editorial. Reports from *General Practice*, 1974, 24.
Stein, P. Some aspects of group practice. *Practitioner*, 1967, *199*, 810-813.
Stevens, J. A brief encounter. The James Mackenzie Lecture, 1973. *Journal of the Royal College of General Practitioners*, 1974, *24*, 5-22.
Vaisrub, S. Playing super-God. *Journal of the American Medical Association*, 1971, *218*, 588.
Wahl, C. W. The physician's treatment of the dying patient. *Annals of the New York Academy of Sciences*, 1969, *164*, 759-775.
Wolfe, S., & Badgley, R. F. The family doctor. *Milbank Memorial Fund Quarterly*, 1972, *50*, Part 2.

Appendix

On General Practice and Family Medicine

It will have been noted by the reader that the terms "general practice" and "family physician" have been used interchangeably. This has been done deliberately but with the result that those who have strong preference as to their titles will probably be offended.

During the course of interviewing physicians, many comments were received about the use of the term "family physician": "it's political," "they're trying to say they're doing something new, but that's not so," "what's wrong with the good old-fashioned title, G.P."

Reference to texts provided little in the way of clues as to the distinction. Knox (1970), writing in Britain, states that:

> the clinical component of general practice is a large one, comprising parts of many disciplines such as general medicine, psychiatry, pediatrics, and many others. . . . The diagnostic process of the general practitioner may follow the same pathway as that of his hospital colleague, but it is further conditioned by such factors as prior knowledge of the normal for a particular patient, his family and his environment (p. 9).

For an initial brief moment, when the two titles are under scrutiny, the word "family" might appear to be the distinction. The College of Family Physicians of Canada, Canadian Family Medicine document (1973) goes into some detail on this matter:

> The physician shall: practice family medicine with the family as the unit of care (3.9), describe the life cycle of the family (3.4), define the role of the family in health care (3.3), use the currently accepted knowledge of individual human development in providing family oriented health care (3.1), be skilled in applying his knowledge of individual and family behavior to the identification and solution of individual health problems (3.6) (p. 75-77).

However, the only real distinction that can be drawn between general practice and family medicine is one that relates not to approach, but to emphasis. Emphasis to what end is the crucial question.

The result may be better quality care, but this has never been proven in a controlled way. More important is that general practice or family medicine now has a new identity in a rapidly changing age. The title family physician allows for specialization without fragmentation and, perhaps for this reason alone, is intuitively attractive.

An actual distinction does not appear to exist, however, and therefore both terms will be used, hopefully without fear or favor!

THE DISCIPLINE OF FAMILY MEDICINE

Collin Baker, MD

There is still a great deal of misunderstanding concerning the significance of the new specialty, family medicine. A considerable body of literature (Committee on Education, AAFP, 1972; Sergent, 1967; Wilson, 1970) has been written on the subject since Haggerty pointed out in 1963 that the old general practice residencies failed precisely because of their failure "to demonstrate decisively what it is that the family physician can do better than the specialist."

The post-Flexner orientation of medical teaching toward the hospital-based academic and research model had several unfortunate consequences in addition to the tremendous technical gains that were made (Janeway, 1974). The fact that teachers in medical schools have been selected, especially in the last 20 years, because of their research potential (and hence their ability to attract grants) has resulted in the almost total exclusion of the general clinician from medical faculties. This, in turn, has caused the generalist to be professionally ostracized and denigrated; it has also encouraged many medical students to turn from their initial orientation toward primary care toward other, more "scientific" careers.

Medical students today are still subject to considerable pressure by their faculty advisors to abandon career goals in primary care in favor of research or the subspecialities. Students tell us of advisors who say "You're too bright to be a family doctor; you would waste your talents," not realizing that to be a competent family physician is one of the most challenging occupations within the medical profession.

It is true that many general practitioners of the past found themselves in a professional blind alley. Following the traditional pattern of solo practice, they frequently were overwhelmed by the constant pressures of patient care which allowed no time for study, recreation, or family. Professionally isolated in many instances, they sometimes failed to keep up with the technical advances which have taken place so rapidly in the last 50 years. Even those who were more fortunately situated found themselves ill prepared to deal with many of the problems that come to the doctor who practices outside the

Dr. Baker is Professor and Director of Undergraduate Programs, Department of Family Medicine, University of South Carolina, Columbia, SC 29208.

Marriage & Family Review, Vol. 4(1/2), Spring/Summer 1981

medical center. Postgraduate training for the family doctor was brief, and until quite recently, it lacked any systematic instruction in the essential skills of the generalist.

Over time and through experience, every good family doctor has developed certain essential capabilities because he has found them necessary to the provision of comprehensive, continuous medical care of high quality in the ambulatory setting. Student physicians previously were not taught these skills in the course of their medical training because the experts in primary care for the family were systematically excluded from the training centers and thus were unable to transmit their skills to oncoming groups of students. As medical training became increasingly hospital-based, training for primary care became more and more unrealistic. It is this failure of medical education that the family medicine movement of recent years is attempting to remedy.

Many family medicine training programs are based in community hospitals, rather than in large teaching hospitals. The advantage is that these hospitals may resemble more closely the sort of environment in which the resident ultimately will practice, and the patient population and the spectrum of disease encountered will provide more realistic opportunities for learning. A teaching affiliation with a nearby medical center or teaching hospital is frequently established to assure that the training is of high quality and to provide periodic evaluation of the training program.

Instead of training residents exclusively in the hospital environment, family medicine training programs now provide for a fourth to a third of all training to be acquired in a model practice setting. This is a training practice which is designed to resemble as much as possible the actual conditions of a private group practice in which the residents deliver health care as members of teams under the preception of family physicians. Some programs give their residents a part of their training in other ambulatory care settings, such as neighborhood health centers.

There is also increased emphasis on experience in the offices of busy practitioners, especially in the second and third years of training. Residents frequently spend from 2 to 6 months of their training time in rural practice; one program devotes the entire second and third years to such training. Quality of care, and consequently of training, are assured by close liaison between the base program and the satellite practice, with frequent evaluations of both residents and preceptors. Preceptors are often encouraged to serve in the model practice on a part-time basis, and exchange programs are being established in which the resident may take the place of a preceptor in a group practice while the preceptor returns to the training program for full-time study and participation in teaching.

Medical students of today are people-oriented, perhaps more than at any other time in history. Many students and some recognized authorities (cf. Eron, 1955) believe that the current process of training physicians is depersonalizing and tends to discourage personal concern for the patient. It seems, instead, to reward the student who develops an impersonal, "scientific" approach to the patient. Whether this is true or not, it is clear to all who are familiar with medical training that there frequently has been a lack of positive teaching regarding the patient as a person with problems who lives in and interacts with a family, in contrast to a person with a disease inhabiting his/her body.

A resurgence of interest in treating the "whole patient" has developed in recent years, perhaps as a part of the public's increasing demand that they have a choice in how they are treated by doctors. Patients appreciate having a physician who can take care of most of their medical problems competently; they understand the need for specialists, but they want to feel that they have an advocate in charge of the total pattern of health care. They want doctors who evince continuous concern for their problems, rather than treat their illnesses episodically. Recognition of these needs of patients is beginning to produce changes in medical education. Student pressures for change in the old, disease-oriented teaching methods are growing. Perhaps most important are the changes in funding sources for medical education which encourage those schools which are really serious about training primary care physicians (Ebert, 1973).

Family doctors with a deep interest in teaching the essential skills that they had to learn for themselves now find themselves back in the medical schools, participating in teaching for the first time in many decades. Their reentry into the academic community did not meet with overwhelming enthusiasm among the academic establishment, as might have been predicted. Besides the matter of turf rights, the newcomers lacked the credentials represented by a clearly-defined area of expertise (McGraw, 1971) and attested to by the publication of papers on research and evaluation in those areas. This deficit has been largely overcome by the emergence of a group of scholars and researchers in family medicine who have built up a considerable literature on the academic aspects of the discipline.

The specific expertise was initially poorly defined because family medicine encompasses the whole patient and all of his/her problems, hence it is impossible to stake out a specialized area of pathology peculiar to the field. It is in other functions, integrative rather than fractionating, that the family doctor excels; these functions are being taught in family medicine training programs throughout the country (Baker, 1974).

The family doctor must be trained to cope with all of the more common conditions seen in ambulatory practice, as well as with the critical and life-threatening emergencies with which he may be faced (Baker, op. cit.). This requires a thorough grounding in internal medicine and pediatrics, both ambulatory and hospital-based. In addition, a good knowledge of office gynecology, orthopedics, otolaryngology, and dermatology is required, as well as an understanding of the principles of surgery and obstetrics. These multiple goals are achievable because no attempt is made to master any one field in its ultimate complexity and detail. This is specialization in breadth, rather than depth.

In family medicine training programs, residents are taught that any problem which affects the health of the patient is within their area of responsibility. They are given the technical capability to treat competently about 95% of the problems with which patients come into the office, and to be aware of the others. They will treat those they can handle best, and will manage by appropriate referral those requiring the services of someone more expert in another field of medicine or in another discipline. Referral of such conditions in no way lessens the responsibility of the physician to continue to be concerned with the patient's problems, and the family doctor continues to follow the patient, acting as advisor in an integrative capacity throughout each illness and beyond.

Referral of problems should not be taken to mean only referral to physicians, but to any other health provider or resource that may help to restore the patient to health. Disease must be considered as anything that impairs the patient's function as a whole person and disturbs his family relationships, and family doctors must be familiar with all the resources of the community which may benefit their patients. They not only must have a good idea of the skills and relative competence of medical consultants, but also must know what agencies and paramedical resources are available to deal with problems of psychosocial origin.

Today's family doctor has better training in the recognition and management of emotional factors in illness, of family conflicts, and of minor psychiatric problems. He learns to integrate the management of these problems into the flow of a busy practice. To facilitate this, he must be trained in the efficient use of ancillary personnel—nurse practitioners, physicians' associates, behavioral science people, and others—so that he can utilize his time optimally for the benefit of his patients.

Great advances have been made in recent years in the design of records for use in the ambulatory setting that make possible greater efficiency in the provision of ongoing, comprehensive care (Cross, 1972; Froom, 1974).

Anyone who has tried to wrestle with the 8-year record of a patient in a typical outpatient department will realize that such improvements are long overdue. Without adequate and concise records, results of tests are lost, diagnostic work is repeated unnecessarily, drug incompatibilities are overlooked, and patients receive multiple prescriptions for the same medications.

Trainees in family medicine programs also learn that the efficiency of their offices is directly related to the effectiveness of their care, and they are trained in the actual management of a medical office–personnel problems, fiscal matters, and supply problems. The lack of training of this kind in the past has contributed both to poorer care and to higher medical costs, yet until recently there has been no attempt to teach these skills to doctors.

Since family physicians are responsible for the health of the whole family through the years, they must be concerned with the prevention and early detection of disease. Preventive medicine in its most personal sense is the province of the family doctor, and strong emphasis is placed on it in training. As better data is accumulated on the real incidence of disease in the ambulatory setting (which was not previously available), family physicians are better able to assess risk factors and to advise their patients of the measures which offer to each of them the best hope of staying well. No longer are complete routine physicals done at the arbitrary interval of 365 days, but the interval and the type of screening examinations done are determined on the basis of the risk represented by the patient's family history, occupation, past medical history, and other factors (Frame & Carlson, 1975). The result is a tremendous saving in medical manpower, plus lower costs and better opportunities for the patient to improve his prospects for good health.

These are the areas of expertise which set the family doctor apart from specialists in other fields. This is not to say that some of these skills are not taught in other training programs; they are, and they should be. But family medicine programs, to a greater degree than any others, have integrated these several skills, developed perforce by family doctors in the past, into a training program that prepares the young doctor for delivery of primary health care in a way that is not duplicated in any other field. This is the discipline of family medicine.

REFERENCES

American Academy of Family Practice. *Education for family practice.* Report of Committee on Education, 1972.

Baker, C. What's Different about Family Medicine? *J. Med. Educ.*, 1974, *49*, 229.

Cross, H. D. The Problem-oriented system in private practice in a small town. In Hurst & Walker (Eds.), *The problem-oriented system.* New York: Medcom Press, 1972.

Ebert, R. H. Biomedical research policy–A reevaluation. *New England Journal of Medicine*, 1973, *289*, 348.

Eron, L. D. Effect of medical education on medical students' attitudes. *J. Med. Educ.*, 1955, *30*, 559-566.

Frame, P. S. & Carlson, S. J. A critical review of periodic health screening using specific screening criteria. *J. Fam. Prac.*, 1975, *22*, 9-36, 123-126, 189-194, 285-288.

Froom, J. The problem-oriented medical record. *J. Fam. Prac.*, 1974, *1*, 48.

Haggerty, R. J. Etiology of the decline in general practice. *Journal American Medical Association*, 1963, *185*, 179.

Haggerty, R. J. General practice–Extinction or rebirth? *Harvard Med. Alumni Bulletin*, 1963.

Janeway, C. A. The decline of primary medical care: An unforeseen consequence of the flexner report. *The Pharos*, 1974, 74-80.

McGraw, R. M. Trends in medical education and health services–Their implications for a career in family medicine? *New England Journal of Medicine*, 1971, *285*, 1407.

Sergent, J. A. Family medicine–An emergent specialty. *Journal American Medical Association*, 1967, *200*, 1158.

Wilson, V. E. Family medicine–Pioneer or slave to the past. *American Family Physician*, 1970, *1*, 131.

FAMILY MEDICINE IN CANADA

J. Ivan Williams, PhD

The Decline of the General Practitioner

The health care system in Canada has been influenced by the following trends of the 1950s and 1960s which have affected health care in most industrialized countries:

1. The explosion of medical knowledge.
2. The rapid expansion of hospital beds and the construction of new hospitals.
3. The development of medical specialties.
4. The relative decline of general practitioners, particularly in the 1950s.
5. Increased costs in health services.
6. Fragmentation and depersonalization of health services.
7. The growing consumer concern for improved availability and access to medical care.
8. Expansion of medical education programs.
9. The increase in medical technology.
10. The increase in chronic care needs.
11. Increased government expenditures in research training programs and health care services.

Under the British North America Act of 1867, the provinces were delegated the responsibility of providing health services, save for those who come under the direct jurisdiction of the federal government (the people in the territories, veterans, treaty Indians). Government involvement came first in public health

---

Dr. Williams is Director of the Health Care Research Unit, Associate Professor in the Department of Health Administration, and Lecturer in the Department of Family and Community Medicine at the University of Toronto, FitzGerald Building, Toronto, Ontario M5S 1A1.

The author would like to express his appreciation to Donald I. Rice, Ian R. McWhinney, and Brian K. E. Hennen for their comments and suggestions. In addition, Donald I. Rice, the Executive Director of the College of Family Physicians of Canada, provided data from the college registry and information about recent actions taken by the College.

The author is solely responsible for interpretations of the information and errors in fact.

Marriage & Family Review, Vol. 4(1/2), Spring/Summer 1981

services, mental health services, and services for the chronically ill and disabled. Public support for medical care and hospital services initially came in the form of assistance of the medically indigent. By World War II, the federal government became increasingly concerned about the disparities in the availability of health services and manpower, and there was a search for a mechanism to reduce the disparities. The National Health Grants Program, established in 1948, provided a series of conditional, cost-sharing grants whereby municipalities and provinces would agree to the terms of the grants and receive funds. The grants allowed for a rapid expansion of general and mental hospital beds, extension of public health services, and increased training opportunities for health personnel.

In 1957, the federal government enacted the Hospital and Diagnostic Services Act of 1957, another conditional, cost-sharing program which provided for universal coverage of hospital services. As capital costs were largely guaranteed by the National Health Grants and as the service costs were guaranteed by public insurance, the hospital increasingly became the focus of the medical care system.

The medical schools were still responding to the criticisms of the Flexner report and they were intent upon training medical scientists. The percentage of physicians in speciality practice increased from 23.1% in 1947 to 51.1% in 1961 (Judek, 1964).

Medical schools faced an additional problem of failing to provide an adequate supply of physician manpower. In 1945 there were nine medical schools, with only two (Manitoba and Alberta) west of Ontario. By the mid-1950s, the University of Ottawa, the University of British Columbia, and the University of Saskatchewan were producing medical graduates (Judek, 1964). Even with the expansion of medical education facilities, the number of medical graduates per population of 100,000 remained relatively constant at about 4.5. During the first half of the decade the ratio of medical students declined from 25.4 per 100,000 persons in 1950 to 22.7 in 1957, and from 1957 to the early 1960s the absolute number of medical students declined as the medical schools were having difficulty in finding qualified applicants (Judek, 1964). Students with strong science backgrounds were pursuing careers in science per se.

There would have been a decline in the physician population ratio in the 15 years following the war had there not been a net migration of physicians. During this time about 5,000 physicians immigrated and about one-half that number emigrated, principally to the United States (Note 1). About one-half (1,764) of the physicians immigrating between 1953 and 1961 were from the United Kingdom and another 471 came from the United States (Judek, 1964).

As Kendall (1971a) has noted, the increase in technology, the growth of medical knowledge, the demands for medical research, the increase in hospital beds, the demands for training facilities, and the demand for medical educators have been trends which have led to specialization and a relative decline in general practitioners, though not a decline in their absolute numbers. As a consequence of the trend toward specialization, there have been other declines experienced by general practitioners (Kendall, 1971b).

In relation to the specialists, they suffered declines in income and prestige. Furthermore, in urban areas specialists began to compete with general prac-

NUMBER AND RATIO TO POPULATION OF ACTIVE PHYSICIANS
CANADA, 1901 - 1974

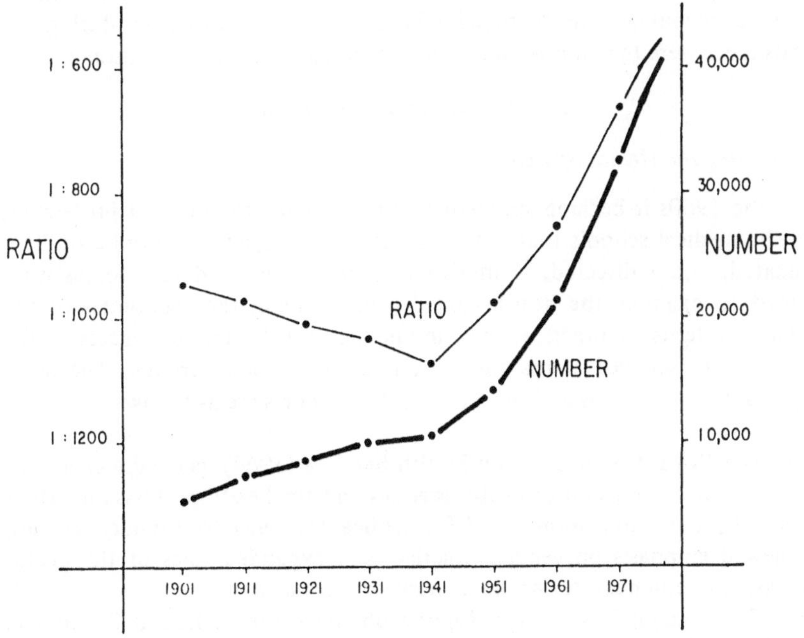

SOURCE: Health Manpower Planning Division, 1973
Health Information Division, 1978

FIGURE I

titioners for patients and they began to question privileges for the general practitioner in the larger city hospitals. The challenge was intensified when Clute (1963) published his study which criticized the quality of care delivered by samples of general practitioners in Ontario and Nova Scotia.

As Freidson (1970) has noted, the medical profession maintains its autonomy by controlling work conditions, the content of practice, and professional education. In order to maintain autonomy, the professional bodies had to meet the challenges which adversely affected half of the physicians in Canada. In the early 1950s the Executive Council of the Canadian Medical Association (CMA) established a working party to study the problem of general practice. As a result of the recommendations, the Council of the Canadian Medical Association formed the College of General Practice of Canada in 1954 for the purposes of upgrading the profession and the quality of primary care. Toward this end, the College stressed the development of continuing education programs in the medical schools, and general practitioners were encouraged to participate in the programs. However, during the 1950s there were few improvements in the status of general practitioners.

The Rise of Family Physicians

Redirecting the Health System

In the 1960s it became apparent to governments, the medical profession, and the medical schools that the entire health care system had to be studied, evaluated, and redirected. Commissions, committees, and task forces were formed to examine the health care delivery system, the economics of the system, patterns of practice, and the unequal distribution and access to the medical care services across the various socioeconomic groups. The more important study groups and the dates of their reports are as follows:

1. The Royal Commission on Health Services (1964), generally called for expansion and extension of health services and the health professsions. More specifically the commission called for medical insurance for primary services, a renewed emphasis on general practice, and expanded roles of the health profession to compensate for the manpower shortages.
2. The Federal Task Force Reports on the Costs of Health Services in Canada (1970) stressed mechanisms for the reduction of costs, particularly in hospital utilization.
3. The Ontario Committee on Healing Arts (1970) placed an emphasis on primary care, on social planning of health services, and for public control of the health professions.

4. The Quebec Commission on the Inquiry into Health and Welfare (1970) called for the functional integration of health and social services, regional organization of services and manpower, and the establishment of Local Health Centers (community health centers) as the fundamental unit in the health care system.

5. The Community Health Center Project Report (1972) called for the integration of medical and health professions working in teams to provide comprehensive primary care in community health centers.

6. The Nova Scotia Council of Health (1972) called for a regional organization of health services with a renewed emphasis on primary care.

7. The Manitoba White Paper on Health Policy (1972) stressed regional organization of health services and the formation of community health centers providing health and social services.

8. Richard Foulkes, in his report on Health Security for British Columbia (1973), called for a radical reorganization of health services with regionalization and community health centers as the key principles.

9. The Ontario Health Planning Task Force (1974) called for the province to be organized into regions and districts, the formation of district health councils for planning and coordination, and the formation of area service management boards to govern both the primary and secondary levels of care. The report calls for centers with teams of health professionals. This report more than any other reflects the logic of the reorganization of health services in England.

The thrust of these commissioned studies was to refocus the medical care system around primary care in the community. There have been moves to reduce utilization of hospital beds by expanding outpatient services in outpatient departments and by expanding diagnostic, follow-up, and home care services in the community.

Within the emphasis of care in the community, there have been incentives and encouragement for, and in some cases the direct endorsement of, the concept of family medicine, which may be defined as the body of medical knowledge related to primary, continuing, and comprehensive medical care to the individual and his family.

Community health centers have been advocated by some planners (Community Health Center Project, 1972), but the relative effectiveness and efficiency of the centers in reducing costs has been questioned (Ruderman, 1972; Williams, 1974; Korcok, 1974). While community health centers have been started in Manitoba, Ontario, Quebec, and Saskatchewan, the federal and provincial governments have not been interested in providing the required capital funding or in reorganizing the patterns of practice of the primary care physicians (Vayda, 1977).

The provincial plans vary in detail, but generally physicians are paid 85% to 90% of negotiated fee schedules, with some provinces permitting the physicans to bill the patients for the uninsured portions. The fee schedules permit specialists to charge higher fees, but some provinces, like Ontario, allow specialist fees only if the patient has been referred by another physician. If specialists treat self-referred patients, they may only recover fees allowable to general practitioners. There have been attempts to reduce the disparities in the fee schedules for services provided by specialists as opposed to the fees paid to family physicians and general practitioners so as to reduce income differences.

Manpower Trends Since 1960

Following the Royal Commission on Health Services (1964) the prevailing assumptions among health planners were that there were shortages of health manpower in general and of physician manpower, specifically general practitioners. Four strategies were pursued to solve the shortages.

First, the health manpower training programs were expanded. As a part of this, four new medical schools were added (University of Calgary, McMaster University, Memorial University of Newfoundland, and Sherbrooke University) and the class sizes of existing schools were enlarged. By 1972, there were 5.8 medical graduates per 100,000 people, an increase of 1.3 medical graduates over the 1961 ratio. By 1977 there were 7.3 medical graduates per 100,000, which was a 26% increase over 5 years. The applicant pool increased even more dramatically so that by 1972 one qualified applicant was refused admission for every position in each year's class, and the abundance of qualified candidates continues.

A second strategy was to consider alternative means of organizing health manpower. Group practices (Boan, 1966) and community health centers (Wolfe & Badgley, 1972; Ruderman, 1972; Anderson & Crichton, 1973) have been advocated as means to improving the effectiveness and efficiency of manpower utilization. A third strategy, related to the second, was to consider expanding the roles of nurses to include activities performed by physicians, and considerable emphasis has been placed on the concept of the nurse practitioner (Committee on Nurse Practitioners, 1972).

Last, the federal and provincial governments became more concerned with monitoring health manpower, and consequently a Health Manpower Directorate was created in Health and Welfare Canada to work with its provincial counterparts in studying the flow of health manpower. More specifically, the provincial governments are considering regionalization of health services as a means for redistributing health manpower.

As can be seen in Figure I, there has been a marked increase in physician manpower since 1961. The unexpected increase came from physicians immigrating to Canada and the decline in those emigrating to the United States (physicians emigrating to the United States could be drafted during the Vietnam War). The net migration resulted in there being one immigrant physician for every graduate of a Canadian medical school (Note 2).

With the increases in medical graduates and immigrating physicians from 1963 to 1972, there was a 48% increase in the number of physicians and a 15% increase in population. Between 1972 and 1977 there was an additional 21.2% increase in the number of physicians, as opposed to a 6.8% increase in population. In 1973 and 1974 there were marked increases in the numbers of immigrant physicians and the number of graduates steadily increased from 1,280 in 1972 to 1,704 in 1977.

More recently there has been a debate about a surplus of physician manpower. The debate is emotionally charged, but at least one task force has suggested that a province begin controlling the number of physicians that may practice, particularly in those specialties where there are apparent surpluses (Ontario Council of Health, 1974). Tighter controls have been placed on the numbers of physicians who can immigrate to Canada.

As can be seen in Table 1, 50.6% of all active physicians in 1977 (excluding interns, residents, and physicians not in private practice) were in general, or family, practice. It can be seen that immigrant physicians were slightly more likely to be generalists than specialists. The College of Family Physicians of Canada has estimated that one generalist is needed for 1750 people, and all provinces now meet this standard (Health Information Division, 1978).

There are two problems which continue. Even though the generalists are more evenly distributed than the specialists, rural areas and northern districts tend to be underserviced. Ontario has established an incentive program which has reduced markedly the number of underserviced areas (Copeman, 1973), but the problem continues. The second problem is that general practitioners may lack specialist's credentials but may in fact work as specialists (Harvey & Harvey, 1970). Consequently the 1:1750 ratio is a crude indicator, as it does not adequately suggest that the above problems remain.

The Rise of Family Medicine

In 1962 the government of Saskatchewan introduced public medical care insurance, and this was the first major thrust of a government into governing the terms of work in community medical care. The medical profession went on strike and the strike failed (Badgley & Wolfe, 1967). Since then the

TABLE I

ACTIVE PHYSICIANS[*] IN CANADA BY PROVINCE
BY TYPE OF PRACTICE, WITH PERCENT FOREIGN BORN IN EACH TYPE
1977

	Active Physicians			Family Physician/ General Practitioner			Specialist		
	Total Physicians	Ratio to Population	% Foreign Graduates	% of Total Physicians	Ratio to Population	% Foreign Graduates	% of Total Physicians	Ratio to Population	% Foreign Graduates
Newfoundland	641	881	56.2	67.4	1,308	56.3	32.6	2,703	56.0
Prince Edward Island	137	891	21.2	61.3	1,452	21.4	38.7	2,302	20.8
Nova Scotia	1,187	708	34.0	55.3	1,277	34.7	44.7	1,583	33.0
New Brunswick	723	957	32.6	55.2	1,734	33.3	44.8	2,136	31.8
Quebec	9,525	659	15.5	41.8	1,576	12.2	58.2	1,134	17.8
Ontario	13,076	646	33.0	52.1	1,238	33.6	47.9	1,349	32.3
Manitoba	1,491	694	41.6	52.3	1,327	48.7	47.7	1,456	33.8
Saskatchewan	1,209	781	55.6	63.7	1,226	60.8	36.3	2,150	46.5
Alberta	2,534	764	40.2	54.0	1,414	44.7	46.0	1,662	34.9
British Columbia	4,278	590	36.7	54.0	1,091	35.1	46.0	1,283	38.5
Yukon	25	880	36.0	88.0	1,000	31.8	12.0	7,333	66.7
Northwest Territories	34	1,294	32.4	76.5	1,692	26.9	23.5	5,500	50.0
Canada	34,860	673	30.7	50.6	1,328	32.2	49.4	1,363	29.2

[*] The 1977 data exclude interns and residents. Health Information Division, 1978.

medical profession has accepted a responsibility to work with government and voluntary associations to assure that medical services serve the public interests (Blishen, 1969). However, the medical profession believes that it has the reponsibility of assuring quality medical care through planning, organizing, and providing medical services, and this belief reflects the doctors' doctrine of professional autonomy (Blishen, 1969). Only two provinces have attempted to exclude the medical profession from the planning and organizing of health services, thereby introducing the possibility of public control of the content of work (Note 3).

The medical profession has provided major briefs and position papers to each of the health planning bodies, and representatives of various professional bodies have participated directly in most of the commission. In response to the challenges, the various professional bodies began to change their points of view. In 1962, the College of General Practice refocused its professional perspective. The College believed that in order to produce physicians who would provide primary, comprehensive, and continuous care in a personalized manner and would be involved in community health care, the educational emphasis would have to be on undergraduate training and residency programs. While their emphasis on continuing education is maintained, the College believed that the role model had to be taught if medical students were to pursue primary care as a career. In accordance with the new emphasis the organization was renamed the College of Family Physicians of Canada, hereafter referred to as the CFPC (Note 4).

The CFPC began to work with the Association of Canadian Medical Colleges (ACMC) to encourage the establishment of continuing education, undergraduate, and residency training programs in each medical school. By 1964 each school had a division of continuing education. The College began to work for the establishment of undergraduate programs and teaching departments, even though the College did not formally state its position until 1967 in the document *Training in Family Medicine* (1967).

By 1973 all but two of the schools (Montreal and Manitoba) had formal divisions or departments of General Practice or Family Medicine, and now all medical schools have departments or divisions of family medicine. The departments have worked to introduce medical students to the clinical methods and perspectives of family practice, usually through clinical clerkships. Furthermore, the faculty of these departments have tended to become involved in the teaching of clinical medicine, epidemiology, human behavior, and human development to relate the concepts and principles of these subjects to family medicine. This trend has received government support in Ontario where the Minister of Health has stated that at least one-half of all graduates should become primary care physicians.

With support and encouragement of the CFPC, the University of Calgary and the University of Western Ontario received grants from the Department of National Health and Welfare to establish the first residency training programs in 1966. The College established educational objectives (which are reviewed later) as guidelines by which program proposals were reviewed. All 16 medical schools now have residency training programs.

Initially there were two approaches to the organization of the training experiences of residents in family medicine. One approach was to have the program located in a teaching hospital and to have residents spend most of their time rotating through specialist services. The University of Toronto was the most prominent program which began with this approach (Perkin, 1972). The logic for doing so was to give family physicians status and prestige equal to specialists, to assure they learned recent advances in technology, and to assure that graduates would be able to relate to the consultants and to the hospital.

The second approach was to locate the teaching unit in the community and to center the training experiences there. McWhinney (1972a) has argued that the content of family practice is sufficiently different from hospital medicine that family practice cannot be learned in a hospital. He argues that the discipline of family medicine is best taught in a family practice unit with family physicians providing the clinical instruction.

The CFPC has encouraged the latter approach, and the hospital programs have made changes accordingly. Most hospital programs now provide learning experiences in community-based clinical settings ranging from occupational health units in an industry, to health centers serving Indian reserves.

There have been and continue to be working ties and relationships between physicians and medical education in Canada and in the United States. Consequently the Coggeshall (1965), Millis (Citizen's Commission of Graduate Medical Education, 1966), and Willard (Ad Hoc Committee on Education for Family Practice, 1966) reports have been used in planning changes in medical education. Some faculty in the programs have been active members in the Society for the Teachers of Family Medicine which is based in the U.S. and have been involved in the continuing education sessions of the American Academy of Family Physicians. However, these associations have tended to focus on issues related to the United States medical care system of little relevance to the Canadian scene. Consideration was given to establishing a separate division of the Society of Teachers in Family Medicine in Canada, and the Canadian Society of Teachers in Family Medicine was formed in 1978.

How the teachers of family medicine were to be trained was questioned. In 1977, the Department of Family Medicine of the University of Western Ontario began to offer an MSc in Family Medicine as a teaching and research degree. At McGill University there is a Center for Advanced Studies in Primary Care for established teachers in the discipline. Both of these programs have been funded by the Kellogg Foundation. For the foreseeable future, though, most teachers of family physicians will gain their expertise through varieties of clinical, research, and educational experiences.

For the concept of family medicine to be successful, it has to be adopted by primary care physicians. In the next section the trends in membership in the CFPC are used as an indication of that acceptance.

Family Physicians as Specialists

The CFPC has three categories of active members:

1. An active member is required to have been active in family practice or a graduate of a residency program.
2. A certificant is the person who has passed the examination set by the College.
3. A fellow is an honor conferred by the College on outstanding members.

To maintain their active status, the College requires the members complete 100 hours of approved postgraduate study every 2 years; failure to do so may result in loss of membership.

The success of the new speciality depends in part on the acceptance of the College by practicing physicians. Table II shows the trends in active membership since 1969, and Table III displays the distribution of the members by province.

The membership of the CFCP has increased steadily and in 1974 about 25% or 3,401 of all primary care physicians were active members of the College, and by 1979, 28.2% of primary care physicians were active in the College.

The membership rates have been lowest in Quebec and Newfoundland. In Quebec, the physicians are organized into the Federation of General Practitioners received its charter in 1963, and its chief activities are:

1. Negotiation with the government concerning fee schedules and other conditions affecting practice.

2. Communication at all required levels.
3. Professional assistance and development for its members.

The number of general practitioners declined until the introduction of medical care insurance, and there was an 11% increase in the first year of the program (Le Clair, 1975).

There are two reasons why the College has not been actively involved. Firstly, the College has been largely anglophonic; only within recent years have there been moves to include French in the professional publications and

TABLE II

ACTIVE MEMBERSHIP IN
COLLEGE OF FAMILY PHYSICIANS OF CANADA

	New Fellows	New Certificants	Active* Members	Total ** Membership
1969	47	12	2065	2526
1970	23	107	2210	2604
1971	8	204	2346	2706
1972	24	206	2695	2988
1973	11	224	3177	3401
1974	4	217	3401	3665
1975	11	300	3714	4070
1976	13	354	4082	4336
1977	12	397	4269	4839
1978	15	392	4601	5331
1979	19	360	4987	5502
	191	2773	4987	5502

* Includes Fellows and Certificants

** Includes Associate and Honorary Members

TABLE III

DISTRIBUTION OF ACTIVE MEMBERS OF THE COLLEGE OF FAMILY PHYSICIANS OF CANADA BY PROVINCE, 1974

		Percentage of primary care physicians
Newfoundland	54	15
Prince Edward Island	31	41
Nova Scotia	180	32
New Brunswick	104	29
Quebec	182	6
Ontario	1788	29
Manitoba	190	27
Saskatchewan	148	22
Alberta	289	24
British Columbia	383	19
Yukon	6	30
Northwest Territories	1	4
Out of Canada	45	
CANADA	3401	25

examinations. The inclusion of French is important as all physicians must be fluent in French before they can be licensed in Quebec.

The second reason is that the Quebec Federation has sought to enlist the College in its political negotiations with the government. The College has stressed education and licensure as the *modus operante* for change and has eschewed overt political involvement.

A graduate training program is being established in primary care at McGill University and other educational efforts are expanding. With the increased use of French, the activities of the College in Quebec can be expected to expand.

In Newfoundland, as the Department of Family Practice develops at Memorial University, one would anticipate that the 50-odd general practitioners in the province would become involved in clinical teaching and in the activities of the College.

In Canada, all certification examinations are set by the Royal College of Physicians and Surgeons (RCPS), save for the CFPC. The CFPC sets its own examinations which consist of written tests, simulated patient interviews with examiners observing through a one-way mirror, and an oral defense. To be eligible for the exam a candidate must be a graduate of an approved residency training program or be practice eligible. A practice-eligible candidate must have been in practice for 5 years, be an active member of the CFPC, and have completed 250 hours of approved postgraduate study in the 5-year period. The College hopes to discontinue practice eligibility by 1980. The new policy dictates that physicians graduating after 1980 can only become eligible by completing a family medicine residency program, but medical students, interns, and residents have protested against this policy as being an undue restriction of career opportunities.

Table IV shows the trends in certification procedures. Canada had approximately 17,654 physicians in active general or family practice in 1977, and 11.4% (2,012) were certified. Of those who were certified, nearly 90% met the practice eligibility criteria. As certification gains acceptance, the proportion of primary care physicians who are certified should increase. It should be noted that the physicians do take a risk in writing the examinations, as one-fourth fail to be certified.

At present there are few incentives for a physician to write the examination. The following structural changes have been considered:

1. Certified family physicians could have schedules of fees higher than general practitioners. The CFPA has considered this mechanism, but has not recommended it because physician income is a contentious political issue and general practitioners could be unnecessarily threatened by this gesture.

2. Hospital privileges of general practitioners are being restricted in some areas, particularly cities, while the privileges of family physicians are not. This action depends upon the medical staff of a given hospital and is not a profession-wide measure.

3. Teaching appointments in family medicine are increasingly being limited to certified family physicians, and this serves to deny a source of prestige and status to general practitioners.

4. Licenses for general practitioners could be limited as recommended by the CFPC.

The General Council of the Canadian Medical Association has recommended that the license to practice be limited to the individual's training and demonstrated competence. With the support of the Association of Canadian Medical Colleges (ACMC) in January 1974, the CFPC recommended to the Federation of Provincial Medical Lincensing Authorities (FPMLA) that only graduates of 2-year residency programs—with 1 year spent in family medicine—be eligible for unrestricted licenses to practice family medicine. General practitioners would have limited licensure which would mean they work under supervision for some types of procedures.

The Royal College of Physicians and Surgeons (RCPS) initially opposed the recommendation since residents may be deterred from specialty training

TABLE IV

CERTIFICATION IN THE

COLLEGE OF FAMILY PHYSICIANS OF CANADA

	Practice Eligible	Percent Certified	Residency Eligible	Percent Certified
1969	7	100.0	6	83.3
1970	110	90.0	12	66.7
1971	273	68.5	20	85.0
1972	246	74.0	31	77.4
1973	208	82.2	59	89.8
1974	205	75.6	76	81.6
1975	243	77.0	133	86.5
1976	212	79.8	193	96.4
1977	229	73.3	236	92.8
1978	204	77.0	268	87.7
1979	196	71.9	258	84.9
TOTAL	2,133	76.5	1,292	88.5

if they cannot receive a full license after dropping from the specialty program before completion. The Canadian Association of Interns and Residents (CAIR) opposed the recommendation because they did not want to see the length of time in training increased and they were concerned the measure might limit their "moonlighting" activities while in training. In addition, the value of the residency program has been questioned. In family medicine the social, emotional, and preventive components of illness and health care are stressed as a part of developing a holistic perspective in primary care. Some students, interns, and general practitioners believe that the rotating internship teaches basic clinical skills and that the added year of training in family medicine is directed to "quasi-psychiatry" rather than to medical science, making the second year unnecessary.

In January of 1975 the CFPC met with representatives of RCPS, CAIR, ACMC, CMA, and the Medical Council of Canada. Within the previous year the Alberta College of Physicians and Surgeons had moved to require 2 years of postgraduate experience prior to licensure. After a debate of the above points of view, the representatives voted to recommend to the FPMLA that the 2-year period of residency–with 1 year in family practice–be required for independent licensure.

Should this recommendation be accepted by the FPMLA and implemented by each provincial College of Physicians and Surgeons, family medicine will have the force of legislative authority behind it. This would mean that residency training programs would have to be expanded from the present 400 positions to about 700 positions. Secondly, there should be a rush of practice-eligible candidates to write the certification examination before the proposed 1980 date of implementation.

The possible responses of the provincial ministries of health to the recommendation are not clear. There would be increased training grants to support the expansion of the residency programs, and they can anticipate a demand for increased fee schedules based on the new levels of competency. At the same time it is not clear that family physicians provide better quality care than general practitioners. The position of the provincial governments could be made more difficult if there were decided splits in the medical profession over the recommendation.

Until there are additional incentives for becoming specialists in family medicine, probably 50% or less of the primary care physicians will be certified. One could also predict that CFPC will continue the practice-eligible criteria for certification until the reward system is restructured to provide more specific incentives and until there are sufficient residency training opportunities for the required numbers of family doctors.

The Content and Practice of Family Medicine

The substance of family medicine can be defined in terms of its content and practice. The content of knowledge is found in the educational objectives of the CFPC. The practice of family medicine is defined by comparing it conceptually with other types of practice.

The Educational Objectives of Family Medicine

The College of Family Physicians of Canada has formed a Committee on Educational Objectives. The Committee outlined seven general objectives, and then restated each of these objectives in increasingly more specific behavioral terms. The College has prepared two booklets, the first of which is related to the performance of family physicians (CFPC, 1973a). The second booklet specifies the content of the body of knowledge that comprises the discipline of family medicine (CFPC, 1973b). The final set of objectives is to be used to structure the curricula of family medicine programs and to evaluate the changes in the knowledge, attitudes, and skills of medical students, residents, and physicians.

The seven basic objectives are outlined in Figure II. The following summary statements indicate some of the areas which are emphasized.

1. Family medicine is to provide primary, comprehensive, and continuing care for the individual and the family. Prevention and health maintenance is stressed as a part of quality medical care.
2. The problem-oriented approach is stressed in assessment and treatment. Social, emotional, and medical problems are to be evaluated from the standpoints of the individual and the physician.
3. A basic understanding of individual and family behavior is to be employed in identifying and solving problems. The life cycle is the basic behavioral science perspective used.
4. An understanding of health care organizations, ranging from the organization of the particular practice and team to the community and national health care systems, is required.
5. The physicians are encouraged to engage in clinical, epidemiological, and health services research. The medical record is viewed as the key to research, and the Problem-Oriented Record developed by Weed is advocated.

It is unclear the extent to which family physicians meet these objectives or put them into practice. Williams and associates (1974) reported on the

FIGURE II

THE EDUCATIONAL OBJECTIVES OF THE COLLEGE OF FAMILY PHYSICIANS OF CANADA

1. The physician shall be skilled in the definition of health problems.
2. The physician shall be skilled in the management of health problems.
3. The physician shall use the currently accepted knowledge of the family providing health care.
4. The physician shall organize his practice efficiently and effectively to provide family care.
5. The physician shall understand and accept the responsibilities of a professional as he practices medicine.
6. The physician shall be able to evaluate the results of research in health care and its delivery, and incorporate them into his practice.
7. The physician shall consider health maintenance as a part of his professional responsibility.

behavioral science content in the residency training programs in Canada and in the United States up to 1972 and found that while most programs included the behavioral sciences, the coverage was not sufficiently comprehensive to meet the objectives.

Even though most teaching units began, and in some cases continue to be, divisions of epidemiology or community medicine, the units almost solely rely upon family physicians as teachers. One can wonder if family physicians who are teachers have sufficient training to be able to teach the broad range of subject matter required to meet the educational objectives. It appears that as the residency training programs develop and stabilize, conceptual seminars are organized, and outside faculty or specialists are brought in to teach particular subject matter to the residents.

Even if behavioral science, epidemiology, health services, and research concepts and principles are taught, residents may be slow to assimilate the concepts and principles as they may be judged irrelevant to family practice.

Both the faculty and the residents may be slow to make basic materials relevant to clinical practice. The practical obstacles to implementing the objectives have not been completely solved.

A Comparative Analysis of Family Practice

In Figure III the practice patterns of family physicians are compared with those of specialists (primary, secondary, and tertiary), public health nurses, and social workers, both in terms of orientation to care and in places of practice. The public health nurses and medical social workers were included as they are increasingly involved in teaching units which train residents in family practice and in primary care settings.

In Canada, the general practitioners and family physicians are generally the physicians of first contact and the sources of comprehensive and community care. In larger urban centers, obstetricians, pediatricians, and internists provide primary and continuing care to individuals who are self-referred. Secondary and tertiary specialists are less likely to have a holistic orientation, in comparison to family physicians, and few specialists of any type have interests in providing family care or in caring for individuals without regard to age, sex, or type of initial problem. There is a minor debate in family medicine as to whether physicians should only accept individuals without their families. The reactions of the public are making the first alternative untenable as individuals do not want their choices of personal physicians restricted by the decisions of family members.

Family physicians and general practitioners have offices in the community and admission privileges in general hospitals. In smaller hospitals in rural areas, the general practitioners perform surgical and medical procedures. Primary specialists have offices in the community and general hospital appointments. Unlike family physicians, specialists deliver almost no domiciliary care. Secondary and tertiary specialists are more likly to confine their practices to hospitals but few hospitals have geographical, full-time positions so that the specialists continue to maintain offices.

Harvey & Harvey (1970) found that physicians who leave general practice for specialty practice have done so because they were unprepared to handle the broad range of problems. Also, the former general practitioners felt they were unable to shape their practices because of heavy patient demands. There has been consideration given to limited licensure to restrict and to redefine the practices of family physicians and specialists, but so far there has been little definitive action. Family physicians would limit their practices to primary, comprehensive and continuing care and would refer patients requiring specialist procedures. They would maintain hospital privileges to perform the

FIGURE III

A COMPARATIVE ANALYSIS OF PRACTICE PATTERNS

	Orientation to Care				
	Primary - Self referral or doctor referred for care	Comprehensive Care for all Problems of Individual	Comprehensive Care for all Problems of Family	Continuing Care for Initial	Continuing Care for All Problems
Family Physicians	self-referred	yes	yes	yes	yes
Primary Specialists[1]	self and doctor referred	generally yes for those self-referred	seldom	yes	sometimes
Secondary Specialists[2]	doctor referred	no	no	yes	no
Tertiary Specialists[3]	doctor referred	no	no	no	no
Public Health Nurse	self-referral and referred	yes	yes	yes	yes
Medical Social Worker	referred	varies	no	yes	no

	Place of Practice			
	Home	Office	General Hospital	Tertiary Service
Family Physicians	sometimes	yes	yes	no
Primary Specialist	no	yes	yes	no
Tertiary Specialists	no	sometimes	yes	yes
Public Health Nurse	yes	yes	sometimes	sometimes
Medical Social Worker	seldom	yes	yes	yes

1. Primary specialists are internists, pediatricians and obstetricians.
2. Secondary specialists are surgeons and psychiatrists.
3. Tertiary specialists are the most highly specialized physicians.

more routine medical procedures and obstetrical care. Under limited licensure specialists would be limited to procedures within their spheres of competence and training.

Public health nurses, both in terms of orientation to care and in place of practice, complement the work of family physicians by more systematically extending care into the community and the home. Social workers offer a broad range of services but they continue to be office based, unless they are interested in community organization. Most social workers in primary care settings either work as counselors or as coordinators of social services. As long as the payment for primary care is based on fees for physician services it is unlikely that public health nurses and medical social workers will be widely employed in the offices of family physicians.

Wolfe & Badgley (1973) argue that if family doctors work in group practices, they can employ public health nurses and social workers to cope with some of the social, emotional, and routine problems that can consume the doctor's time. By working with other family doctors, individual doctors can focus, in part, on particular types of patients or problems that are of interest.

There are arguments that economics of scale are achieved in group practice (Boan, 1966; Bailey, 1970). However, the evidence is mixed. In his review of studies, Kaufman (1976) indicates that physicians in group practice provide more services per physician than in solo practice, but there is little evidence to suggest that group physicians see more patients than their counterparts in solo practice. Group practices may generate more services and income per physician than do solo practices, but they apparently do so by increasing the average costs of health care per patient. While the gross income per physician may increase for group practices, group physicians tend to have greater total expenses than solo practitioners so that the differences in net income by type of practice are minimal (Ruderman, 1972). The intangible benefits of group practice appear to be greater than the economic ones.

General practitioners in England are offered substantial financial incentives to relocate in community health centers and to work under the aegis of district health councils. Until there are stronger incentives for family physicians to reorganize practice patterns, one can expect them to be slow to change, just as their counterparts in England have been.

Summary and Conclusions

The decade of the 1950s was a period of decline for general practitioners and general practice. In the decade of the 1960s there was considerable effort and attention given to the refocus and redirection of the health care system. The main emphases have been to functionally integrate services and to reestablish the community as the locus of the system.

Beginning in the 1960s and continuing to the present, the medical profession in general, and the College of Family Physicians of Canada in particular, have been developing the discipline of family medicine to be taught in medical schools, family practice as a new way to organize care, and specialty recognition for family physicians to implement the discipline and practice.

The trends in government policy, medical education and medical manpower were reviewed, and the content and practice of family medicine were conceptually analyzed. To this point the development of family medicine has been determined largely by members of the profession who have voluntarily participated to upgrade themselves, to rebuild the reputation of primary care, and to improve the quality of practice.

There are four structural changes in the medical care system which could enhance the status of family physicians. Family physicians could bill on a higher fee schedule than general practitioners. Secondly, the general practitioners could have more restricted hospital privileges than family physicians. Thirdly, general practitioners could be excluded from teaching appointments. Lastly, general practitioners could be granted a license to practice under supervision while family physicians would be granted unlimited licenses. The CFPC is advocating differential licensure for family physicians over general practitioners but it is not clear whether doctors' organizations and provincial governments will accept the recommendation.

Even though the concept of family medicine has made tremendous gains in the past decade, one can question whether most primary care physicians will become involved in the movement until there are structural incentives for changing their practice and for refocusing their professional orientation. Family medicine can be expected to survive and to thrive as a voluntary movement, but it is doubtful whether it will predominate professional perspectives of primary care physicians until there are additional changes in the health care system.

NOTES

1. There was an interestingly anomoly in the medical schools. Over one-third of the medical students at McGill University were from the United States, and most returned after graduation. This pattern was followed until the university had to rely heavily upon provincial funding, at which time the percentage of students from the United States dropped markedly.

2. There are two basic criticisms of the high rate of physician immigration. Firstly, reliance upon immigrants means that Canada is not training its own citizens for high status positions. Secondly, the Third World countries have been critical of Canada and the United States for accepting scarce medical manpower from countries that can least afford the loss. Because of these two concerns and the concern about a surplus, the federal government recently tightened immigration policies to make it more difficult for physicians to immigrate.

3. Quebec and Manitoba are the two provinces which have questioned whether the associations could serve the public while pursuing professional interests. In Quebec the professions are now governed by lay bodies and in both Quebec and Manitoba the professional associations are considered to be collective-bargaining agents and hence are excluded from health planning. The specialists started to strike in Quebec, but they were forced to abandon their plans by the general practitioners' support of the government, by the labor movement's opposition, and by the October crisis in 1970. The striking specialists were largely anglophones who encountered strong opposition from the francophones. The Manitoba Medical Association (1972) challenged the White Paper of the socialist government (New Democratic Party) and threatened to strike, though no action was taken. Since then the Progressive Conservative Party formed the government, and the White Paper was set aside.

4. Family medicine refers to the discipline, family practice refers to the organization of primary services, and family physicians are the specialists who put the discipline into practice. McWhinney (1972b) suggests that the term "general practice" is outdated because:

1. It is increasingly difficult for doctors to engage generally in all types of medical practice.
2. It is difficult to view general practice as a body of knowledge of discipline.
3. The term continues to carry negative connotations among academic physicians and others.

General practitioners argue that years of tradition should not be so easily discarded and that the term be redefined to reflect the new patterns of practice. Hence, both sets of definitions are used and the debate continues. Two academic departments carry the name General Practice but the journal *Canada Family Physician* discourages the use of the traditional terms in its articles.

REFERENCES

Ad Hoc Committee on Education for Family Practice of the Council on Medical Education. *Meeting the challenge of family practice*. Chicago: American Medical Association, 1966.

Anderson, D. O., & Crichton, Anne O. J. *What price group practice*? Vancouver: University of British Columbia, 1973.

Badgley, R. F., & Wolfe, S. *Doctor's strike: Medical care and conflict in Saskatchewan*. Toronto: MacMillan Company of Canada, 1967.

Bailey, R. M. Economics of scale in medical practice. In H. E. Klarman (Ed.). *Empirical studies in health economics*. Baltimore: Johns Hopkins Press, 1970, 255-273.

Blishen, B. R. *Doctors and doctrines: Ideology of medical care in Canada. Toronto, University of Toronto Press, 1969.*

Boan, J. A. *Group practice: Royal commission on health services*. Ottawa: Queen's Printer, 1966.

Citizen's Commission on Graduate Medical Education. *The graduate education of physicians*. Chicago: AMA, 1966.

Coggeshall, L. T. *Planning for medical progress through education*. Chicago: Association of American Medical Colleges, 1965.

College of Family Physicians of Canada. *Training in family medicine*. Don Mills, Ontario: College of Family Physicians, 1967.

College of Family Physicians of Canada. *Canada family medicine: Educational objectives for certification in family medicine*. Don Mills, Ontario: College of Family Physicians of Canada, 1973.

Committee on the Costs of Health Services. *Task force reports on the costs of health services in Canada* (3 vol.). Ottawa: Department of National Health and Welfare, 1970.

Commission in Inquiry on Health and Social Welfare. *Health*, 1970, *IV*, Quebec City: Government of Quebec.

Committee on Nurse Practitioners. *Reports of the committee on nurse practitioners*. Ottawa: Department of National Health and Welfare, 1972.

Community Health Centre Project. *The community health centre in Canada*. Ottawa: Information Canada, 1972.

Foulkes, R. G. *Health security for British Columbians*. Victoria: Department of Health, 1973.

Freidson, E. *Professional dominance: The social structure of medical care*. New York: Atherton Press, 1970.

Government of Manitoba. *White paper on health policy*. Winnipeg: Department of Health and Social Development, 1972.

Harvey, E. B., & Harvey, L. R. *Ontario medical manpower project* (mimeographed), 1970.

Health Information Division. *Canada health manpower inventory*. Ottawa: Department of National Health and Welfare, 1978.

Health Manpower Planning Division. *Canada health manpower inventory*. Ottawa: Health and Welfare Canada, 1973.

Judek, S. *Medical manpower in Canada. Royal commission on health services*. Ottawa: The Queen's Printer, 1964.

Kaufman, B. *The economics of group practice versus solo practice: A survey paper*. Paper No. 4, Health Care Research Unit, The University of Western Ontario, London, Ontario, 1976.

Kendall, P. L. Medical specialization: Trends and contributing factors. In R. H. Coombs & C. E. Vincent (Eds.), *Psychosocial aspects of medical training*, Illinois: Charles C. Thomas, 1971, 449-497.

Kendall, P. L. Consequences of the trend toward specialization. In R. H. Coombs & C. E. Vincent (Eds.), *Psychosocial aspects of medical training*, Illinois: Charles C. Thomas, 1971, 498-523.

Korcok, M. Community health clinics: Are they cost effective? *Canadian Medical Association Journal*, 1974, *III*, 1347-1351.

Le Clair, M. The Canadian health care system. In S. Andereopoulos, Spyros (Ed.), *National health insurance: Can we learn from Canada*? New York: John Wiley & Sons, 1975, 9-96.

Manitoba Medical Association. *Health care in Manitoba as of today and tomorrow*. Winnipeg: Manitoba Medical Association, 1973.

McWhinney, I. R. Postgraduate programs should emphasize practice of family medicine. *Canadian Family Physician*, 1972, *18*, 83.

McWhinney, I. R. General practice and family medicine. *Canadian Family Physician*, 1972, *18*, 111.

Nova Scotia Council of Health. *A new direction for the seventies*. Halifax, Nova Scotia: Department of Health, 1972.

Ontario Committee on Healing Arts. *Final report*. Toronto: Queen's Printer, 1970, 3 volumes.

Ontario Council of Health. *Physician manpower*. Toronto: Ontario Council of Health, 1974.

Ontario Health Planning Task Force. *Report of the health planning task force*. Toronto: Government of Ontario, 1974.

Perkin, R. L. "Vicarious experience" school: A defense. *Canadian Family Physician*, 1972, *18*, 17-18.

Royal Commission on Health Services. *Final report*. Ottawa: Queen's Printer, 1964, 2 volumes.

Ruderman, A. P. *Economic characteristics of community health centre project*. Ottawa: Information Canada. 1972.

Vayda, E. Prepaid group practice under universal health insurance in Canada. *Medical Care*, 1977, *15*, 382-389.

Williams, J. I. Community health centres: Unanswered questions. *Canadian Consumer*, 1974, *4*, 4-7.

Williams, J. I., Bishop, F. M., Hennen, B. K. E., & Johnson, T. W. Teaching of behavioral sciences in family medicine residency programs in Canada and the United States. *Social Science and Medicine*, 1974, *8*, 565-574.

Wolfe, S., & Badgley, R. F. *The family doctor*. Toronto: MacMillan Co. of Canada, 1972.